MEDIUM ÆVUM MONOGRAPHS

EDITORIAL COMMITTEE

K. P. Clarke, A. J. Lappin,
N. F. Palmer, P. Russell, C. Saunders

MEDIUM ÆVUM MONOGRAPHS
XXXII

CONTEXTUALIZING MIRACLES IN THE CHRISTIAN WEST, 1100-1500

NEW HISTORICAL APPROACHES

EDITED BY MATTHEW M. MESLEY AND LOUISE E. WILSON

The Society for the Study of Medieval Languages and Literature

OXFORD · MMXIV

THE SOCIETY FOR THE STUDY OF
MEDIEVAL LANGUAGES AND LITERATURE

OXFORD, 2014

http://mediumaevum.modhist.ox.ac.uk

© The Authors, 2014

Cover design by Richard Rowley

British Library Cataloguing Publication Data
A catalogue record for this book is
available from the British Library

ISBN-13: 978-0-907570-24-0 (hb)
ISBN-13: 978-0-907570-32-5 (pb)

CONTENTS

Matthew Mesley 1
    Introduction

Anne E. Bailey 17
    Peter Brown and Victor Turner Revisited:
    Anthropological Approaches to Latin Miracle
    Narratives in the Medieval West

Simon Yarrow 41
    Miracles, Belief and Christian Materiality: Relic'ing
    in Twelfth-Century Miracle Narratives

Kati Ihnat 63
    Marian Miracles and Marian Liturgies in the
    Benedictine Tradition of Post-Conquest England

Louise Elizabeth Wilson 99
    Conceptions of the Miraculous: Natural Philosophy
    and Medical Knowledge in the Thirteenth-Century
    Miracula of St Edmund of Abingdon

Iona McCleery 127
    'Christ More Powerful Than Galen'? The
    Relationship Between Medicine and Miracles

Irina Metzler 155
    Indiscriminate Healing Miracles in Decline: How
    Social Realities Affect Religious Perception

Rebecca Pinner 177
    St Edmund of East Anglia: 'Martir, Mayde and
    Kynge', and Midwife?

Fiona Kao 197
    John Foxe's Golden Saints? Ways of Reading Foxe's
    Female Martyrs in Light of Voragine's *Golden Legend*

The Contributors 229

INTRODUCTION

Matthew M. Mesley

And the pope thanked God that it pleased him to show such miracles for his holy martyr, at whose tomb by the merits and prayers of this holy martyr our blessed Lord hath showed many miracles. The blind have recovered their sight, the dumb their speech, the deaf their hearing, the lame their limbs, and the dead their life. If I should here express all the miracles that it hath pleased God to show for this holy saint it should contain a whole volume ...

The Golden Legend: St Thomas of Canterbury.[1]

During the middle ages both the laity and clergy recognized that miracles were signs of God's intervention in the world. Indeed, it is no exaggeration to say that miracles and wonders pervade the thought-worlds and writings of medieval men and women. As with the miracles performed by Jesus in the Bible for the blind and 'demonically possessed', it was through their manifestation that medieval saints were shown to act as conduits of divine will; miracles worked to reveal their sanctity – it was one way that saints demonstrated their holiness to those around them, both during their life and after death. Throughout the medieval period, therefore, pilgrims travelled to saints' shrines in order to seek a miraculous cure or treatment for their various ailments. It was at these shrines or tombs that accounts of miracles were written down in order to provide a recording of a saint's miraculous acts for posterity, and/or to promote the saints of particular institutions; elsewhere, postmortem-miracles continued to be placed at the conclusion of many saints' *vitae* that chronicled their subjects' lives

---

[*] I would like to thank Drs Katherine Lewis, Christopher Bonfield and Louise Wilson for making suggestions on earlier versions of this introduction, and to Dr Anthony Lappin for his comments on an initial draft.

[1] Jacobus de Voragine, *The Golden Legend: Readings on the Saints*, translated by William Granger Ryan, 2nd edn (Princeton, 2012), 59-62.

and great works. Increasingly, from the late eleventh century, *miracula* were produced in specific collections – as Rachel Koopmans put it, after the Norman Conquest 'miracle-collecting mania began to spread'.[2] The reasons and motives for documenting such events were varied; for some it was a way to provide a written account of earlier oral recollections about a community's saint; for other institutions it may have been a response to social, political or local change.[3]

By the late twelfth and early thirteenth centuries authors of such collections and the communities for which they were written, were aware that these accounts could be used as evidence in canonization proceedings, the official process by which the papacy authenticated a saint. Yet, to use England as an example, the papal commissions which would lead to the canonizations of both Gilbert of Sempringham (1202) and Bishop Wulfstan of Worcester (1203), also demonstrated how the decision-making procedures increasingly involved a dialogue between religious communities and the church hierarchy.[4] Furthermore, while miracles were still considered to be an essential component in validating sainthood, the style and structure of texts produced changed as the criteria for canonization was made more rigorous; from the thirteenth century, testimonies and legal depositions, in which the statements of

---

[2] Rachel Koopmans, *Wonderful to Relate: Miracle Stories and Miracle Collecting in High Medieval England* (Philadelphia, 2011), 2.

[3] In responding to Koopmans' work Stephanie Hollis critiqued the author's specific focus: 'Miracle collecting in her view was a literary phenomenon'. In contrast, Tom Licence notes that Koopmans 'is right to challenge the tendency to read politics and propaganda into texts primarily envisaged as devotional exercises'. Perhaps it is best to acknowledge that different texts can be approached in multiple ways. For the reviews see Stephanie Hollis, *Parergon*, 29 (2012), 224-26; and Tom Licence, *American Historical Review*, 117 (2012), 587-88.

[4] See Raymonde Foreville, 'Canterbury et la canonisation des saints au XIIe siècle', in *Tradition and Change: Essays in Honour of Marjorie Chibnall*, edited by Diana Greenway, Christopher Holdsworth and Jane Sayers (Cambridge, 1985), 63-75. And for Gilbert, specifically Michelle Light, 'Evidence of sanctity: record keeping and canonization at the turn of the 13th Century', *Archivaria*, 60 (2005), 105-23. How canonization may have influenced writers of hagiography at the time is also explored briefly in Helen Birkett, *The Saints' Lives of Jocelin of Furness: Hagiography, Patronage and Ecclesiastical Politics* (York, 2010), 211-16.

witnesses and the miracles they had observed were carefully scrutinized, became standard.⁵ As Robert Bartlett has stated, 'hagiography became a legal brief in the literal as well as the metaphorical sense'.⁶ If the earlier variety of miracle accounts remain – that is, those recorded and kept at shrines, or those rewritten for an institutional audience – the fashion for collecting *miracula* slowed to a trickle in the later medieval period. However, miracle narratives persisted and were produced in other contexts; restyled and repackaged, they would be also translated into the vernacular, to be read and appreciated by new, and increasingly diverse, audiences.⁷

*

This volume arose out of a conference at Wolfson College, Cambridge, in April 2011, and reflects on how the study of miracles has transformed over the twentieth and twenty-first centuries.⁸ It aims to unpick and contextualize beliefs about

---

⁵ In specific reference to the relationship between miracles and canonization, see Gábor Klaniczay, 'Speaking about miracles: oral testimony and written record in medieval canonization trials', in *The Development of Literate Mentalities in East Central Europe*, edited by Anna Adamska and Marco Mostert (Turnhout, 2004), 365-96.

⁶ Robert Bartlett, 'Hagiography of Angevin England', in *Thirteenth Century England V*, edited by Peter R. Coss and Simon D. Lloyd (Woodbridge, 1995), 52.

⁷ This is of course a concise synopsis of a vast subject, and many of the contributors look at the scholarship in greater depth. Extensive and significant analyses of miracles and the miraculous by previous scholars have shed light upon medieval conceptions of sainthood, the processes and institutionalization of canonization, and the broader social and cultural attitudes towards saints' cults and miracles. Including but not limited to Eric W. Kemp, *Canonization and Authority in the Western Church* (London 1948); Ronald C. Finucane, *Miracles and Pilgrims: Popular Beliefs in Medieval England* (London, 1977); André Vauchez, *La sainteté en occident aux derniers siècles du Moyen Age: d'après les procès de canonisation et les documents hagiographiques* (Rome and Paris, 1981); Donald Weinstein and Rudolph M. Bell, *Saints & Society: The Two Worlds of Western Christendom, 1000-1700* (Chicago and London, 1982); and Pierre-André Sigal, *L'homme et le miracle dans la France médiévale (XIe-XIIe siècle)* (Paris, 1985).

⁸ In April 2011 the editors convened a conference entitled *Contextualizing Miracles in the Christian West, 1100-1500: New Historical Approaches* at Wolfson College, University of Cambridge. The conference was sponsored

miracles, highlighting their significance in research areas that have hitherto been understudied, and drawing out the methodological implications that arise in extending these avenues of investigation. The main impetus for producing this collection was a recognition by those who participated in the colloquium that in articulating how they encounter and utilize miracles within their work, they were required to rethink their methods of analyzing their texts. In many respects, this volume provided the scholars with a springboard from which to test their theories and engage with the question of the miraculous.

The contributors reflect diverse backgrounds within their field, yet each were united in seeking to consider how we might reorient the way we study miracles. Collectively they ask: how should we analyze the evidence? What tools are available? And how does previous scholarship shape the way we think about, engage with, and interpret the evidence? It represents the work of scholars from various stages in their careers and different specialisms, such as medical history (Iona McCleery, Irina Metzler and Louise Elizabeth Wilson), which has seen a burgeoning interest in miracle narratives; ecclesiastical and social history (Kati Ihnat, Simon Yarrow and Anne E. Bailey) and more literary-based scholars (Rebecca Pinner and Fiona Kao). In addition, researchers who are employing novel theoretical and methodological approaches to their evidence (Yarrow and Bailey) are placed alongside those who adopt more traditional methods of source criticism, where narratives are fruitfully scrutinized and contextualized (Ihnat and Wilson). All these works are distinct and 'stand-alone' pieces of scholarship, yet some common conclusions emerge. Furthermore, the relationship between the texts investigated, the contexts in which they are situated, and the tools employed by the authors, also overlap in important ways. For example, as Yarrow and Bailey clarify, in analyzing narrative representations, consideration of an author's intention or motives is vital; there is always a danger for the scholar in accepting at face value the way authors wanted to represent or symbolize miracles within these texts. Moreover, several of the

by Medium Ævum: The Society for the Study of Medieval Languages and Literature, The Royal Historical Society, and the University of Cambridge, Faculty of History, Doctoral Conference Fund.

chapters draw attention to the attitudes and beliefs of those who were unable to record their experiences; Yarrow and Pinner ask how stories or relics might have interacted with broader audiences, including the illiterate or laity. In so doing they also point to those who had the authority (often clerical or monastic authors) to interpret or explain their significance. As Ihnat suggests, there was a recognition of alternative understandings underpinning certain miracles, and writing down a version of the story (often for an institution, yet not always) provided a powerful means of controlling or prioritizing this interpretation. Even where miracles were not the primary focus of a text, they shed invaluable light on other contemporary ideas, beliefs and practices. As Irina Metzler explores, variations in thinking about those on the periphery of society were reflected in images of the disabled and poor. Miracle stories thus point to the interactions and negotiations between those who had authority to construe meaning, and those who were obliged to accept these views and, more rarely, reject them.[9]

*

The relationship between a text and how a miracle or the miraculous was understood did not remain fixed or unchanged throughout the medieval period. Within Christendom a more systematized 'theology of miracles', which focused upon the mechanisms involved in the miracle event, was developed and

---

[9] Miracles have recently been used to explore perceptions of minorities or relations between religions: for example, Arietta Papaconstantinou, 'Saints and Saracens: on some miracle accounts of the early Arab period', in *Byzantine Religious Culture: Studies in Honor of Alice-Mary Talbot*, edited by Denis Sullivan, Elizabeth Fisher and Stratis Papaioannou (Leiden, 2012), 323-38; and Matthew Mesley, '"*De Judaea, muta et surda*": Jewish conversion in Gerald of Wales's *Life of Saint Remigius*', in *Christians and Jews in Angevin England: The York Massacre of 1190, Narratives and Contexts*, edited by Sarah Rees Jones and Sethina Watson (York, 2013), 238-49. For investigating attitudes to gender and women, see Kathleen Quirk, 'Men, women and miracles in Normandy, 1050-1150', in *Medieval Memories: Men, Women, and the Past, 700-1300*, edited by Elizabeth van Houts (London, 2001), 53-71; Hilary Powell, 'The "Miracle of Childbirth": the portrayal of parturient women in medieval miracle narratives', *Social History of Medicine*, 25.4 (2012), 795-811; Anders Fröjmark, 'Childbirth miracles in Swedish miracle collections', *Journal of the History of Sexuality*, 21.2 (2012), 297-312.

debated in the intellectual arena throughout the course of the middle ages.[10] Attempts (whether by the papacy or specific theologians) to create or impose a more uniform view did not necessarily entail a less complex field of interpretation; nor did it mean that a consensus was actually reached.[11] Understanding the hagiographical and theological conventions that act as a framework for saints' lives and *miracula* has been the point of departure for many of the authors in this volume.[12] However, as Wilson shows in her chapter, theology cannot be isolated from developments in other areas of intellectual thought and practice. This is why we, as editors, have decided to focus upon 'contextualizing' in the title to this volume; thus acknowledging the different environments that influenced beliefs about miracles, along with the variety of textual evidence available and the diverse motives for their production. But more than this, it emphasizes how far the study of miracles is a dialectical process; by engaging with the contexts of both sources and the broader historiography, we can reflect upon what

[10] See in particular Michael E. Goodich, *Miracles and Wonders: The Development of the Concept of Miracle, 1150-1350* (Aldershot, 2007). And also John A. Hardon, 'The concept of miracle from St Augustine to modern apologetics', *Theological Studies*, 15 (1954), 229-57.

[11] This might entail also rethinking how or to what extent miracles should be situated within broader trends. See Steven Justice, 'Eucharistic miracle and eucharistic doubt', *Journal of Medieval and Early Modern Studies*, 42.2 (2012), 307-22.

[12] Writers of saints' lives and *miracula* were keenly aware of their responsibilities in this respect. As Sofia Gajano has commented: 'in hagiographical texts there is a constant concern to establish, or perhaps better, to reestablish, the correct theological relationship, that of the miracle as an external *signum* [sign] of a spiritual holiness that the saint constructs through practicing virtues'. Sofia Boesch Gajano, 'The use and abuse of miracles in early medieval culture', in *Debating the Middle Ages: Issues and Readings*, edited by Barbara H. Rosenwein and Lester K. Little (Oxford, 1998), 335. Useful still is Benedicta Ward, *Miracles and the Medieval Mind: Theory, Record and Event, 1000-1215* (Aldershot and Philadelphia, 1982); and Benedicta Ward, 'Miracles in the middle ages', in *The Cambridge Companion to Miracles*, edited by Graham H. Twelftree (Cambridge, 2011), 149-64. Also, *The Miracles of Our Lady of Rocamadour: Analysis and Translation*, edited and translated by Marcus Bull (Woodbridge, 1999). Bull's introduction is very helpful in surveying the importance of *miracula* in what he terms 'medieval hagiographical culture'. For an approach that explores the literary and theological themes that exist in saints' lives see Michael Staunton, *Thomas Becket and his Biographers* (Woodbridge, 2006).

conceptual frameworks we should use, and how the process itself can enable and extend our understanding of medieval miracles.

Our contributors examine their texts from different perspectives *and* also suggest we should look afresh at the methodological tools we have in our arsenal; in particular, we hope to open up discussion about the need for a diversity of methodological approaches, and stimulate debate about the way we approach miracles as source material.[13] While scholars in the 1970s and 80s sought to quantify and organize the plethora of texts recording miracle accounts medieval scribes produced for the purposes of canonization throughout the high and late medieval period, this collection often addresses avenues of investigation that are situated outside this paradigm. Yet, the legacy of scholarship still shapes the way we think about, engage with, and interpret the evidence. To take one example of how contributors have reflected upon previous historiography, McCleery suggests that 'there is something inherently countable about miracles'; and when used in combination with approaches such as social-statistical methods (what she terms the "bread-and-butter of hagiography"), they can provide an insightful and nuanced tool of analysis. Others in the volume (for example Metzler), focus instead on depictions or themes within miracle narratives collections or stories; such an emphasis can pinpoint specific structures or draw attention to the impact of social and cultural developments on ideas about the miraculous. While Ihnat and Pinner primarily focus upon the institutional and local contexts in which miracles were located or fashioned, Wilson, Yarrow, Bailey and Kao explore the function and interpretation of miracles or hagiographical accounts within particular kinds of texts. They highlight the importance of both literary and oral traditions in shaping how authors represented the miraculous, but they also consider the interplay between authors and readers, the different conventions and particular interests

---

[13] A particularly thoughtful article is Gábor Klaniczay, 'Ritual and narrative in late medieval miracle accounts: the construction of the miracle', in *Religious Participation in Ancient and Medieval Societies: Rituals, Interaction and Identity*, edited by Sara Katajala-Peltomaa and Ville Vuolanto (Rome, 2013), 207-24.

displayed by individual writers, and the meanings and significance of specific accounts, images or retellings.[14]

Bailey opens the collection by suggesting that anthropology is a useful tool in any investigation of miracles and medieval belief.[15] Bailey provides an eloquent and insightful overview of how anthropological methods were applied in earlier debates, and how structural functionalism influenced the conclusions these historians drew. Moreover, she argues that criticism of earlier approaches often gave tacit approval to a certain policing by scholars of the interpretive tools and the texts we examine. Bailey demonstrates that, by applying a 'ritual reading' as a form of textual analysis, we can think about how miracle narratives were themselves efforts to construct specific ideals about the Christian community – who its members were, who had authority, and who could interpret the miraculous?[16] Using twelfth-century miracle narratives she highlights how we can utilize the approaches advocated influentially by Peter Brown and Victor Turner if we redeploy their methods constructively. We can thus ask different questions of the material: not only what the texts tell us about medieval society or life *per se*, but instead at how they reveal patterns of thinking about

---

[14] Such relationships have been explored by a number of earlier scholars: Julia M.H. Smith, 'Oral and written: saints, miracles, and relics in Brittany, c. 850-1250', *Speculum*, 65 (1990), 309-43; Simon Yarrow, 'Narrative, audience and the negotiation of community in twelfth-century English miracle collections', in *Elite and Popular Religion*, edited by Kate Cooper and Jeremy Gregory, Studies in Church History, 42 (Woodbridge, 2006), 65-77; Koopmans, *Wonderful to Relate*.

[15] A number of our contributors have used anthropological methods to good effect in their previous studies: see Simon Yarrow, *Saints and their Communities: Miracle Stories in Twelfth-Century England* (Oxford, 2006); Irina Metzler, *Disability in Medieval Europe: Thinking about Physical Impairment during the High Middle Ages, c. 1100-1400* (London, 2006); and Anne E. Bailey, 'Modern and medieval approaches to pilgrimage, gender and sacred space', *History and Anthropology*, 24.4 (2013), 493-512.

[16] A useful critique still is Philip Rousseau, 'Ascetics as mediators and as teachers', in *The Cult of Saints in Late Antiquity and the Early Middle Ages: Essays on the Contribution of Peter Brown*, edited by James Howard-Johnston and Paul Antony Hayward (Oxford, 1999), 45-59. In particular his comment (51): 'Any judgment on the 'function' of the holy man must take into account the function of the texts. Successful analysis depends on assessing the role configured, not just within the anecdote, but by the very nature of the text itself'.

miracles and illuminate the assumptions medieval hagiographers made or sought to convey. As such, 'rituals-within-the-text' highlight how the author created his or her identity in relation to the miraculous.[17]

In the second chapter, Yarrow asks if medievalists might 'get beyond belief'? It is a question that other medievalists have raised before.[18] But Yarrow's method of tackling this problem is to explore how relics within miracle narratives provide a way of considering whether saints' cults offered medieval people opportunities to transform the meaning of objects. One of functionalism's most rooted legacies, he explains, has been the two-tier interpretation of religious culture – the neat division of contemporaries into 'elite' and 'popular' perspectives. Yarrow shows that the strength of this model was partly derived from literate contemporaries who rhetorically paid lip-service to this dichotomy; it allowed them to shut down any interpretation of events which did not follow the *litterati's* authoritative sanction.[19] With relics, Yarrow argues, we have a way out of this impasse. The manner in which pilgrims interacted with objects and the material culture of a cult, was often expressed differently from what authors sought to promote or encourage. Indeed, using these items men and women outside the clerical sphere imposed values or associations which drew upon more than an acceptance of Christian tenants, or of approved channels of devotion or piety.[20]

---

[17] Although critiqued by many, a still useful exploration of the relationship between authorial intent and ritual is Philippe Buc, *The Dangers of Ritual: Between Early Medieval Texts and Social Scientific Theory* (Princeton, 2001).

[18] Susan Reynolds, 'Social mentalities and the case of medieval scepticism', *Transactions of the Royal Historical Society*, sixth series, 1 (1991), 21-41; and John Arnold, *Belief and Unbelief in Medieval Europe* (London, 2005).

[19] A dichotomy that has much traction even in the last decade: see a number of the titles in *Elite and Popular Religion*, edited by Kate Cooper and Jeremy Gregory, Studies in Church History, 42 (Woodbridge, 2006).

[20] Referring to the theories of a number of scholars, Caroline Walker Bynum states 'what religion – lived religion – does is to lift ordinary objects, in ways consonant with what they are *as objects*, into special significance that makes them conduits of power' in her *Wonderful Blood: Theology and Practice in Late Medieval Northern Germany and Beyond* (Philidelphia, 2007), 48. For another approach to material objects within texts, see Philippe Buc, 'Conversion of objects: Suger of Saint-Denis and Meinwerk of Paderborn', *Viator*, 28 (1997), 99-144.

If Yarrow draws attention to what authors of miracle accounts might have wished to remain concealed, Ihnat seeks to explain the deliberate inclusion of liturgical material in post-Conquest Marian miracle collections.[21] In her detailed and compelling study she explores the juxtaposition and use by Anglo-Norman monastic writers of liturgy and ritual observances within miracle and hagiographical narratives. In the main Ihnat shows how specific liturgies were used to redirect and bolster Marian devotion within particular monastic communities. She argues that miracles can be read simultaneously as a broader response to institutional developments and social pressures, and to intellectual debates over the status of Mary, which took place throughout Europe at this time.[22] Ihnat's piece suggests again that medievalists need to be willing to move beyond their comfort zones, and acknowledge that miracle stories or narratives were not insulated from other forms of cultural forms and artifacts. In the case of liturgies, we see how they interacted with, and were embedded within the miraculous.

Wilson's chapter is a cogent analysis of the miracle collections of the saintly archbishop of Canterbury, Edmund of Abingdon (d. 1240). The 'grand narrative' which explains how the concept of the miraculous was redrawn and reformulated in the thirteenth century is shown in a more complex light when approached from a perspective that interrogates specific manuscript contexts and the terminology employed by different authors. Wilson's study links a number of developments in natural philosophy, theology and medicine, all of which impacted upon how hagiographers described and recounted saintly cures, as well as the ways in which they explained illness, disabilities and death. Her novelty is in revealing how the authors she studies were not simply responding to the

---

[21] An example of incorporating liturgy into studies of monastic communities is Susan Boynton, *Shaping a Monastic Identity: Liturgy and History at the Imperial Abbey of Farfa 1000-1125* (Ithaca, 2006).

[22] Research on Mary is extensive, but in respect of its impact on hagiography and literature see Adrienne Williams Boyarin, *Miracles of the Virgin in Medieval England: Law and Jewishness in Marian Legends* (Cambridge, 2010); and Gary Waller, *The Virgin Mary in Late Medieval and Early English Literature* (Cambridge, 2011). A useful starting point is Miri Rubin, *Emotion and Devotion: The Meaning of Mary in Medieval Religious Cultures* (Budapest and New York, 2009).

conditions that canonization necessitated. Her chapter clarifies how writers of miracle accounts had access to an extensive vocabulary, and made use of scholastic concepts in their explanations of the miraculous in order to make connections and add verisimilitude to their claims. Yet, their use of ideas drawn from different areas of contemporary thought were still interwoven with the topoi and motifs from conventional hagiography. As with Ihnat's piece on the influence of liturgy, here we see how concepts not typically associated with hagiographical literature became assimilated into accounts of the miraculous.

Implicit in Wilson's analysis is a warning against being inhibited by a particular perspective; recognizing that we should keep an open mind about the evidence, and not use material in a way which forces it to fit our modern classifications. This is made explicitly clear by our next contributor, McCleery. Her chapter, set outside medieval England, provides a unique insight into the way scholarship on miracles so often brings with it a certain conceptual baggage about the categories employed. The target of McCleery's scholarly ire is the delineation of the 'spheres' of medicine and the miraculous. In problematizing the concept of 'medicine' and by highlighting that we need to jettison the dichotomy of 'religion' and 'medicine' as two stable categories, she demonstrates how miracle narratives reproduced and contributed to a matrix of contemporary ideas about healing, treatment and spiritual care. In exploring three Portuguese saints' cults dating between the thirteenth and fifteenth centuries, and adopting a perspective not previously applied to these or comparative sources, she demonstrates how historians of medicine can employ miracle accounts and narratives more fruitfully in their studies. Indeed, McCleery's chapter provides important insights into contemporary notions about the body, and how people responded to illness and their recovery.[23] Furthermore, in focusing on Portugal, where no formal canonization process existed until the early modern period,

---

[23] Recent work on healing miracles includes Robert Bartlett, *Why Can the Dead do Such Great Things? Saints and Worshippers from the Martyrs to the Reformation* (Princeton, 2013), 349-64. And see also Gábor Klaniczay, 'Healing with certain conditions: the pedagogy of medieval miracles', *Cahiers de recherches médiévales et humanistes*, 19 (2010), 235-48.

she provides a useful counterpoint to a resilient Anglo or Francocentric paradigm, which, too often, views late medieval saint-making solely in the light of canonization. The emphasis upon canonization procedures, while understandable due to the volume of evidence which these processes produced, can limit our understanding of saints' cults and miracles by concentrating our attention solely on top-down perspectives and 'official' accounts. There is also one element of her cogent argument that others should take away and deliberate, and that is the following assertion: medicine 'in these narratives is a form of religion'; how might this change our way of thinking about miracles?[24]

If we can pinpoint a growing medicalization of society in the later medieval period, albeit with a careful understanding of what this implies, what impact did this have upon perceptions of the miraculous? Metzler highlights how such a process needs to be understood in relation to a variety of societal developments. In particular, Metzler argues that what constituted a 'proper miracle', and who were deemed worthy of such miraculous cures, changed subsequent to the thirteenth century. The late-medieval religious landscape saw a reduction in the number of recorded healing miracles, and a shift in emphasis from thaumaturgic miracles to those of a more spiritual function. Metzler links this to changing ideas about who was considered worthy of the saints' intercessory powers. A number of factors were involved in these changes; first, as the concept of 'voluntary poverty' became increasingly attractive as a spiritual model, in part due to the popularity of the Friars, those deemed poor by fate rather than choice were now considered unsuitable recipients of God's mercy and his miracles. Secondly, the rise of other forms of religiosity, marked by the promotion of asceticism and bodily mortification, in turn produced a loss of status for those who were already physically or mentally impaired.

---

[24] Such an argument chimes with the opinions of medical historians such as Carole Rawcliffe and Peregrine Horden (in particular, their work on the 'medicine of the soul' offered in medieval English hospitals). See Carole Rawcliffe, *Medicine for the Soul: The Life, Death and Resurrection of an English Medieval Hospital* (Stroud, 1999); Peregrine Horden, 'A non-natural environment: medicine without doctors and the medieval European hospital', in *The Medieval Hospital and Medical Practice*, edited by Barbara S. Bowers (Aldershot, 2007), 133-46, at 141.

Men and women who, through their vocation or social status, had cultural and religious capital, could inflict harm or pain upon their bodies for spiritual growth; it was these people who were now deemed to be far more worthy of miraculous intervention. What is clear is that a variety of circumstances influenced contemporary beliefs, ranging from the popularity of institutions, such as the chantries that provided more palatable ways of gaining spiritual rewards, to increased fears about the untrustworthiness of 'fraudulent beggars'. As with other contributors, Metzler illustrates how the task of contextualizing the miraculous entails more than a familiarity with the 'religious domain'. A whole host of economic, cultural and social trends contrived to regulate who was and who was not viewed as worthy enough to receive miraculous intervention.

One of the many frustrations inherent to investigating miracle narratives is appreciating that a text only provides a partial reflection of any given cult. These official representations, mediated through the motives of an author or a community's needs, omit much of how cults could be perceived outside their institutional focal point.[25] It is with these considerations in mind that Pinner studies the representation of St Edmund of East Anglia's cult throughout the middle ages, demonstrating how his 'saintly identity' had different meanings in a variety of settings. Pinner argues that in order to appreciate the characteristics and contours of a cult, we have to explore the interaction between the official and the marginal. She begins with the curious case of an antiphon of St Edmund's, which was performed during the labour of Queen Eleanor of Provence, wife of Henry III, and teases out the gendered connotations of this ritual performance. Here Edmund's portrayal was provided with a different gloss from that presented by the monks of Bury St Edmunds. But by examining the language used to describe the saint in the surviving textual traditions, and

---

[25] To use one example, Elisabeth van Houts has shown how monastic and clerical men were more reluctant to accept the authenticity of female witnesses to miracles. Elisabeth van Houts, *Memory and Gender in Medieval Europe 900-1200* (Basingstoke, 1999). On the possibility of lay agency see Carl S. Watkins, 'Religion and Belief', in *A Social History of England, 900-1200*, edited by Julia Crick and Elisabeth van Houts (Cambridge, 2011), 265-89, from 284-89.

exploring his local and regional significance, the use of the antiphon becomes more explicable. What at first might seem like an anomaly, actually provides an insight into what those outside the monastery's walls desired from their saint. Pinner's reasoned piece is in part a rejoinder to a historiography that often prioritizes the view from the cloister, or eschews evidence that cannot be situated within a preconceived narrative.

Kao's chapter on John Foxe's (d. 1587) female martyrs provides a fitting conclusion to this collection. Working on sixteenth-century material, Kao demonstrates that the conventional identification of texts as either 'medieval' or 'early modern' is in fact an artificial division. In her analysis of Foxe's martyrologies, she shows that not only did his representation of female martyrs echo his own confessional sentiments, they also reflected his debt to late medieval hagiography. Kao's analysis demonstrates how this Protestant polemicist cherry-picked and reused motifs and topoi from a variety of medieval texts, adapting them to specific accounts, to meet his purposes, and to match his audience's presumed expectations. Foxe possessed an ambivalent attitude to the miraculous, one which actually reflected a legacy from pre-Reformation writers, who were often critical of superstitious or credulous beliefs; earlier commentators have been hesitant in tracing such continuities. Analyzing accounts of three female Reformation martyrs (Rose Allin, Joyce Lewis and Mrs Prest), Kao highlights that while Foxe wished to show his subjects as heirs to the classical martyrs of late antiquity, the nature of his revisions were at times far closer to his medieval Catholic predecessors. Even if situated within a 'Reformed context', the continuities that existed between Foxe and the earlier writers of medieval hagiography are striking, and complicate our notions both of periodization, and of how writers of the premodern world represented saints, martyrdom and the miraculous.

Throughout this collection of essays a number of common themes, arguments and intersections emerge. While clarifying how their own work has benefitted from previous scholarship, the contributors suggest that at times the assumptions implicit within earlier historiography have set the agenda, limited the area of scope, or certain questions have been taken for granted; methodologically too, a number of the scholars attempt to move beyond the comfort of stable binaries; 'religion' and 'medicine'; 'high' and 'popular' culture. This collection highlights how miracles in the medieval world might be extraordinary and otherworldly, but they could also be familiar, and associated with the routine and mundane of medieval life. When attempting to describe and analyze medieval society, the miraculous can be deceptively perceived as a vestige, evidence for which can be used to demonstrate the unquestioning credulity of the vast majority of medieval people, relevant only to the pre-modern world. Miracles are sometimes portrayed in ways that are comparable to the subjects of earlier orientalists: there is a tendency to highlight the exotic, the fantastic or the irrational, even when today miracles are believed by millions of religious observers.[26] This is perhaps the reason why miracles are at times only examined or situated within the 'religious sphere', insulated from socio-cultural ideals and practices;[27] yet as this collection highlights, the miraculous was never solely characterized in ways that were isolated from other beliefs, rituals, philosophies and trajectories.[28] In part, if these essays are about contextualizing the evidence we have, they are also about inserting the miraculous back into the broader trends and developments of the medieval world, and analyzing the relationships they had with such processes. Ultimately, the volume as a whole seeks to extend our understanding of the miraculous in the medieval west, to integrate the study of the topic into wider historical study and to re-examine the assumptions of previous generations of scholars, presenting new approaches and contexts to the miraculous in medieval Europe.

---

[26] See, for instance, Robert A. Scott, *Miracle Cures: Saints, Pilgrimage, and the Healing Powers of Belief* (Berkeley, 2010).

[27] In thinking of miracles as part of a wider cultural edifice, the following work has been useful: David L. D'Avray, *Medieval Religious Rationalities: A Weberian Analysis* (Cambridge, 2010).

[28] Similar approaches have been made to saints' cults and hagiography. One example is Katherine Lewis, 'History, historiography and re-writing the past', in *A Companion to Middle English Hagiography*, edited by Sarah Salih (Cambridge, 2006), 122-40.

PETER BROWN AND VICTOR TURNER REVISITED: ANTHROPOLOGICAL APPROACHES TO LATIN MIRACLE NARRATIVES IN THE MEDIEVAL WEST

Anne E. Bailey

> One of the greatest dilemmas bedevilling attempts to unravel the medieval miracle story has been the difficulty distinguishing fact from fiction and imagination from reality.[1]

This chapter explores the past contribution, and future possibilities, of social and cultural anthropology as an approach to miracle narratives in the medieval West. With particular reference to the work of Peter Brown and Victor Turner, it begins by discussing the impact of Durkheimian ideas on the way in which saints' cults, pilgrimage and miracle stories have been understood and studied by medievalists since the 1970s. The chapter continues by turning to the models of twentieth-century ritual theorists such as Victor Turner and Claude Lévi-Strauss, and suggests how scholars might usefully re-deploy these conceptual tools for textual analysis. Drawing on examples of miracle stories produced in twelfth-century England, it argues that a 'ritual' reading of hagiographical narratives offers both a fresh interdisciplinary approach to saints' cults and miracles, and a reassessment of the relationship between fact and fiction in hagiographical texts.

A volume dedicated to the topic of medieval miracles attests to the enormous popularity of the subject with scholars over the last thirty years. However, this flourishing area of research is a relatively recent phenomenon. Before the late 1970s there was a notable dearth of 'miracle' scholarship due, mainly, to post-Enlightenment

---

[1] Michael E. Goodich, *Miracles and Wonders: The Development of the Concept of Miracle, 1150-1350* (Aldershot, 2007), 1.

attitudes towards the miraculous.² Advocates of the 'scientific method' in the eighteenth and nineteenth centuries had not considered hagiography to be a bone fide historical source, and historians such as Edward Gibbon famously poured scorn on medieval people who 'foolishly' believed in miracles.³ Although the Bollandists began preserving hagiographical material from the seventeenth century, a major shift in attitudes was heralded by the appearance of Hippolyte Delehaye's *Lés legends hagiographiques* in 1905.⁴ Nonetheless, 'scientific' attitudes towards medieval saints and miracles were clearly difficult to shake off.⁵ Even Ronald Finucane's pioneering book, *Miracles and Pilgrims: Popular Beliefs in Medieval England*, still makes Gibbon-like references to 'credulous people' and 'gullible clerics'.⁶ In this respect, it is perhaps not all that surprising that Finucane should have chosen a deliberately 'scientific' and 'factual' approach to miracles himself. In *Miracles and Pilgrims*, Finucane turned to the social sciences – specifically sociology and anthropology – as a means of validating a hagiographical source viewed so suspiciously by previous generations.⁷

---

[2] Ronald Finucane and Benedicta Ward popularised the study of miracle collections with seminal works on the subject in 1977 and 1987 respectively. Ronald Finucane, *Miracles and Pilgrims: Popular Beliefs in Medieval England* (London, 1977); Benedicta Ward, *Miracles and the Medieval Mind: Theory, Record and Event, 1000-1215* (Philadelphia, 1987).

[3] Thomas J. Heffernan, *Sacred Biography: Saints and their Biographers in the Middle Ages* (Oxford, 1992), 55-57. Gibbon described the middle ages as an 'age of superstition and credulity', and labeled believers of miracles as 'primitive Christians' and 'ignorant rustics'. Edward Gibbon, *The History of the Decline and Fall of the Roman Empire*, edited by David Womersley, volume 3 (London, 1994), 94, 95, 97, 428.

[4] *Les légendes hagiographiques* (Brussels, 1905) was translated into English in 1962: Hippolyte Delehaye, *Legends of the Saints*, translated by Donald Attwater (London, 1962).

[5] Even Delehaye expressed frustration at hagiography's 'lack of probity'. Heffernan, *Sacred Biography*, 57.

[6] Finucane, *Miracles*, 30, 55. It is instructive to compare Finucane's vocabulary with that of Gibbon: for example, the words 'ignorance', 'credulity' and 'rustics' figure in both. For Edward Gibbon, see note 3 above.

[7] Finucane's statistical methodology, which allowed him to formulate general theories on the numbers, sex, social backgrounds and motivations of visitors to medieval shrines, was taken from anthropological studies of pilgrimage. This approach to miracle collections has since proved popular with

Finucane's book enjoyed success due, in part, to the fact that it struck a chord with the historiographical trends of the time: in the 1970s and 1980s historians were actively looking to the social sciences for new interpretative approaches. The social science method which found particular favour with scholars like Finucane had originally been popularised by the French sociologist Émile Durkheim. In his seminal work, *The Elementary Forms of Religious Life*, Durkheim offered historians a way around post-Enlightenment 'belief' issues by effectively re-inventing religion as a social phenomenon. This was a radical intellectual mind-shift which placed religious belief within an acceptable empirical framework. Under the umbrella of the social sciences with its Durkheimian emphasis on 'fact', religious practices which had so discomforted past historians were now imagined as 'social institutions' fulfilling socio-cultural needs.[8] This approach, structural-functionalism, was adopted by social historians in the 1970s. Although by no means the only scholarly approach to medieval saint devotion, structural-functionalism has, to a large extent, influenced the ways in which medievalists have engaged with the cult of saints and miracle stories ever since.[9]

---

medievalists: see, for example, Pierre-André Sigal, *L'Homme et le miracle dans la France médiévale: XIe-XIIe siècle* (Paris, 1985); John M. Theilmann, 'English peasants and medieval miracle lists', *The Historian*, 52 (1990), 286-303; Eleanora C. Gordon, 'Child health in the middle ages as seen in the miracles of five English saints, AD 1150-1250', *Bulletin of the History of Medicine*, 60 (1986), 502-22; Irena Metzler, *Disability in Medieval Europe: Thinking about Physical Impairment during the High Middle Ages, c. 1100-1400* (London, 2006), 126-85; Sharon Farmer, *Surviving Poverty in Medieval Paris: Gender, Ideology and the Daily Lives of the Poor* (Ithaca and London, 2002); *The Miracles of St Æbbe of Coldingham and St Margaret of Scotland*, edited and translated by Robert Bartlett (Oxford, 2003), xxiii-xxv; Anthony Lappin, *The Medieval Cult of Saint Dominic of Silos* (Leeds, 2002), 97-113; Stanko Andrić, *The Miracles of St John Capistran* (Budapest, 2000), 299-350.

[8] For sociological phenomenon as 'social fact', see Émile Durkheim, *The Rules of Sociological Method*, translated by Sarah A. Solovay and John Henry Mueller (Glencoe, Illinois, 1938). For another discussion of the evolution of secular functional theory, see Philippe Buc, *The Dangers of Ritual: Between Early Medieval Texts and Social Scientific Theory* (Princeton and Oxford, 2001), 161-247.

[9] A useful discussion of the pros and cons of functionalist strategies versus the pro and cons of socio-historical techniques which focus on 'historically valid data', can be found in Marcus Bull, *The Miracles of Our Lady of Rocamadour: Analysis and Translation* (Woodbridge, 1999), 11-20.

Peter Brown: Structural Functionalism and the Cult of Saints

Peter Brown is best known for his work on the religious culture of late-antique and early-medieval Europe, and for situating local religious institutions, such as holy men in the East and saints in the West, within their contemporary political and social structures.[10] Brown was heavily influenced by the work of Émile Durkheim and his interpretation of religion as a social process.[11] In *The Cult of the Saints: Its Rise and Function in Latin Christianity*, Brown enthusiastically embraced Durkheim's sociological approach, and framed saints' cults as collective communities, in which the cult 'centre' (represented by the saint) and its clients (the saint's devotees) were bonded together through ties of interdependence and reciprocity. In this way, Brown demonstrated that saints' cults had a social and political function, in addition to a religious one, in western Europe between the third and sixth centuries.[12] The structural-functionalism espoused by Brown proved popular with other medievalists. Not only did it provide new insight into the relationship between saints' cults and society, but it also gave scholars a useful conceptual tool with which these could be framed. Moreover, Brown's model was found to be as applicable to twelfth-century England as to fifth-century Gaul.[13]

Brown's adoption of structural-functionalism was also instrumental in another way: it allowed him to formulate a revisionist approach to 'popular' religion. Before the 1970s, the

---

[10] See, for example, the essays in Peter Brown, *Society and the Holy in Late Antiquity* (Berkeley, 1982), and Peter Brown, 'The saint as exemplar in late Antiquity', *Representations*, 2 (1983), 1-25.

[11] Brown makes explicit his debt to Durkheim in Brown, 'Saint as exemplar', 12.

[12] Peter Brown, *The Cult of the Saints: Its Rise and Function in Latin Christianity* (Chicago, 1982).

[13] Scholarship particularly influenced by this approach includes Henry Mayr-Harting, 'Functions of a twelfth-century shrine: the miracles of St Frideswide', in *Studies in Medieval History Presented to R. H. C. Davis*, edited by Henry Mayr-Harting and Robert I. Moore (London, 1985), 193-206; Simon Yarrow, *Saints and their Communities: Miracle Stories in Twelfth-Century England* (Oxford, 2006); Susan J. Ridyard, 'Functions of a twelfth-century recluse revisited: the case of Godric of Finchale', in *Belief and Culture in the Middle Ages: Studies Presented to Henry Mayr-Harting*, edited by Richard Gameson and Henrietta Leyser (Oxford, 2001), 236-50.

cultural mentality of the illiterate majority was often conceptualised as standing in structural opposition to that of the religious elite. However, in *The Cult of the Saints* Brown resolved the popular/elite dialectic by arguing that ordinary people shared the beliefs of their religious leaders. According to Brown, the saint's shrine represented a place where all society was united into what he called 'a greater whole', functioning – until the thirteenth century – through popular 'consensus'.[14] Again, this social model has been applied by medievalists, and miracle collections compiled in western Europe are often seen as products of communal collaboration and integration.[15]

Brown's reappraisal of the 'popular' versus 'elite' dichotomy brought with it a heart-warming picture of Christian solidarity and social cohesion, as Simon Yarrow has also noted in this volume. But is such a model a convincing reflection of social reality? A comparison of scholarship produced by medievalists and anthropologists working on saints' cults in their respective fields is instructive. At a time when medievalists tended to view their cults in terms of 'collaboration', and 'negotiating communities', anthropologists had moved into a postmodern phase, and were referring to modern cults in terms of 'conflict' and 'contestation'.[16] Ethnographical studies in the late twentieth century frequently focused on pilgrim diversity, and on clashing aims and desires.[17] In

---

[14] Brown, *Cult*, 12-22. Brown argued that a shift from 'consensus' to 'authority' occurred between the eleventh and twelfth centuries: Peter Brown, 'Society and the supernatural: a medieval change', *Daedalus*, 104 (1975), 133-51.

[15] For example, in her chapter on miracle stories, Leigh Ann Craig repeatedly uses phrases such as 'consensus memory', 'community consensus', 'collaborative authorship' in claiming that miracle stories were 'the product of a collaborative storytelling effort'. Leigh Ann Craig, *Wandering Women and Holy Matrons: Women as Pilgrims in the Later Middle Ages* (Leiden, 2009), 85, 87, 88, 89, 90, 95, 97, 98, 105, 109, 111, 114, 116, 121.

[16] For a discussion of this trend in anthropology, see Simon Coleman, 'Do you believe in pilgrimage? *Communitas*, contestation and beyond', *Anthropological Theory*, 2 (2002), 355-68.

[17] Michael J. Sallnow, 'Pilgrimage and cultural fracture in the Andes', in *Contesting the Sacred: The Anthropology of Christian Pilgrimage*, edited by John Eade and Michael J. Sallnow (London, 1991), 137-53; Jill Dubisch, *In a Different Place: Pilgrimage, Gender and Politics of a Greek Island Shrine* (Princeton, 1995), 219-22; Michael J. Sallnow, '*Communitas* reconsidered: the sociology of Andean pilgrimage', *Man*, 16 (1981), 163-82; John Eade,

short, the shrine was imagined as 'an arena of competition and struggle', rather than as a place representing co-operation and synthesis.[18] This cross-discipline comparison raises an interesting methodological question. Are these disparities due to real differences between the medieval and modern worlds, or can they be explained in terms of contrary interpretative trends?

As an argument for the latter, we might note that a corrective to the collaborative approach has been tested by Barbara Abou-el-Haj. Her 1991 article, 'The Audiences for the Medieval Cult of Saints', draws attention to the fact that saints' cults were not always quite as 'functional', nor as harmonious, as some modern commentators might have us believe. In one of a handful of examples, Abou-el-Haj looks at evidence for the cult of St James at Santiago de Compostela. While the hagiographical *Codex Calixtinus* depicts the cult as a 'spectacle of structured social integration', a very different story seems to have been given by the contemporaneous *Historia compostellana*: one of mob violence and factionalism. Abou-el-Haj concluded that much medieval hagiography was built around 'fantasies of consensus'.[19]

There seems some justification, then, for claiming that the notion of saints as community-bonding forces might be something of a hagiographical construction. Indeed, if we carefully read between the lines of miracle narratives, many of these texts indicate the presence of heretics, witches and doubters who attempted to disrupt the communal harmony.[20] Twelfth-century miracle

---

'Order and power at Lourdes: lay helpers and the organization of a pilgrimage shrine', in *Contesting the Sacred: The Anthropology of Christian Pilgrimage*, edited by John Eade and Michael J. Sallnow (London, 1991), 51-76; Robert Hertz, 'St Besse: a study of an Alpine cult', in *Saints and their Cults: Studies in Religious Sociology, Folklore and History*, edited by Stephen Wilson (Cambridge, 1983), 55-100; Simon Coleman, 'From England's Nazareth to Sweden's Jerusalem: movement, (virtual) landscapes and pilgrimage', in *Reframing Pilgrimage: Cultures in Motion*, edited by Simon Coleman and John Eade (London, 2004), 45-68.

[18] Sallnow, 'Pilgrimage and cultural fracture', 143.

[19] Barbara Abou-el-Haj, 'The audiences for the medieval cult of saints', *Gesta*, 30 (1991), 3-15. For a similar approach to early medieval hagiography, see Buc, *Dangers of Ritual*, 37-157.

[20] Michael E. Goodich, 'Miracles and disbelief in the late middle ages', *Mediaevistik*, 1 (1988), 23-38; Michael E. Goodich, 'Innocent III and the miracle as a weapon against disbelief', in *Lives and Miracles of the Saints:*

collections, for example, are full of stories of vociferous troublemakers who encourage bystanders to join in with the ridicule of a local saint. In one example, a youth is shown entertaining a crowd by placing a white hen on St Ivo's altar and standing on one leg in mock imitation of a cripple.[21] The frequency of such stories in twelfth-century collections suggests that the relationship between cult centres and local communities was often less than harmonious, and such stories are invariably couched as salutary warnings, with their protagonists suitably punished by the judgement of God. In the case of St Ivo's denigrator, we learn that he became crippled himself and spent the remainder of his days living out the condition he had so rashly lampooned. We might, then, argue that the reason that miracle narratives lend themselves so readily to functional analysis is because their hagiographers promoted the notion of successfully functioning cults, an idea also touched upon by Simon Yarrow in this volume.

However, understanding miracle narratives as 'fantasies of consensus' does not necessarily devalue structural-functionalism as an analytical tool. Although some scholars have questioned the validity of employing anthropological strategies in medieval contexts, I would argue that structural-functional theories can be profitably adapted to interpret the structure and function of medieval narratives, and to illuminate the socio-religious objectives of hagiographers.[22] Moreover, because consensus and social cohesion are said to be the main functions of religious ritual, this provides the possibility of a more nuanced structural-functional approach to miracle narratives.[23] We might read these stories as a

---

Studies in Medieval Latin Hagiography, edited by Michael E. Goodich (Aldershot, 2004), 456-71.

[21] Goscelin of Saint-Bertin, *Miracula S. Ivonis*, edited by William D. Macray, Rolls Series, 83 (London, 1886), lxix-lxx.

[22] For an example of a scholar arguing against the deployment of ritual theory, see Philippe Buc in *The Dangers of Ritual*.

[23] The idea of ritual as a community-bonding force was first outlined by Émile Durheim, and lies behind the work of many twentieth-century structural-functionalists such as Alfred Radcliffe-Brown, Bronislaw Malinowski, and Marcel Mauss, and the structuralism of Claude Lévi-Strauss and Mary Douglas. For a more up-to-date take on ritual theory, see Catherine Bell, *Ritual Theory and Ritual Practice* (Oxford, 1992).

type of textual ritual: that is, as written sources which ritually express the consensus 'fantasies' of a collective hagiographic culture. The rest of the chapter will explore some of the possibilities of this alternative approach by re-visiting the ritual theories of some well-known cultural anthropologists, beginning with the ever-popular, but much criticised, work of Victor Turner.

Victor Turner and Pilgrimage

Victor Turner was a British ethnographer whose primary interest lay in the cultural symbols and religious practices of an East African tribe, the Ndembu. Like many cultural anthropologists of his time, Turner adapted his ritual theories for universal application. Some of these proved attractive to medievalists, such as his writing on '*communitas*' which has much in common with Brown's notion that saints' cults offered 'moments of unstructured meeting' to Christian devotees.[24]

However, it was with his best-selling book, *Image and Pilgrimage in Christian Culture*, that Turner particularly came to the attention of medievalists.[25] Borrowing a structural model from the French anthropologist Arnold Van Gennep, Victor and Edith Turner likened Christian pilgrimage to a 'rite of passage'. The generic term 'rite of passage' (*rite de passage*, alternatively translated 'rite of transition'), denoted any ritual which marked an individual's transition from one social status to another. Through three distinct phases, rite-of-passage initiates were ritually separated from, and then re-united with, human society and established norms. In spatial/temporal terms Van Gennep had coined these stages 'pre-

---

[24] Brown, *Cult*, 43. For '*communitas*', see Victor Turner, *The Ritual Process: Structure and Anti-Structure* (New York, 1995), 94-165; Victor Turner, 'Social dramas and ritual metaphors', in *Dramas, Fields and Metaphors: Symbolic Action in Human Society*, edited by Victor Turner (Ithaca and London, 1974), 52, 45. Compare these to Brown, *Cult*, 41-44. One difference between the ideas of Brown and Turner is that, for Brown, 'concord' ideally united the whole of society, whereas Turner's *communitas* was an experience limited to pilgrims.

[25] Victor Turner and Edith Turner, *Image and Pilgrimage in Christian Culture: Anthropological Perspectives* (New York, 1978).

liminal', 'liminal' and 'postliminal'.[26] The Turners adapted this model, and broadened its application to include medieval pilgrimage.[27]

Although remaining popular, Turner's universalising models are frequently criticised for being too abstract and reductionist to be effectively applied to specific real-life experiences.[28] However, this kind of objection becomes less relevant if structural models are applied to a written literary medium, particularly hagiography. Miracle narratives share surprising structural similarities with Turner's rite-of-passage framework, inviting a comparative study. Mapping miracle narratives onto Turner's ritual model may not necessarily add to our knowledge of how medieval pilgrimage was practised but, as will be shown, it can help elucidate the structural thought-worlds of medieval hagiographers and highlight an important sociological function of the miracle genre.

Miracle stories from twelfth-century England seem strangely amenable to a rite-of-passage analysis in a number of ways. Perhaps the most fundamental is that each miracle story is arranged around a three-fold structure which, in the majority of cases, depicts the main protagonist — usually a pilgrim — first departing from, and then returning to, mainstream society. At the most basic level, the majority of pilgrims in the stories fall victim to misfortune, such as sickness or disability, and leave their community to undertake a restorative pilgrimage (Turner's pre-liminal phase). At their destination, pilgrims are shown achieving communion with the divine at the threshold (*limen*) of the spiritual world, literally at the

---

[26] Arnold van Gennep, *The Rites of Passage*, translated by Monika. B. Vizedom and Gabrielle L. Caffee (Chicago, 1960). The Turners summarise this in Turner and Turner, *Image and Pilgrimage*, 1-2.

[27] Turner and Turner, *Image and Pilgrimage*, 172-202.

[28] Criticism is usually directed towards the concepts of *communitas* and liminality. See, for example, Andrea Dahlberg, 'The body as a principle of holism: three pilgrimages to Lourdes', in *Contesting the Sacred: The Anthropology of Christian Pilgrimage*, edited by John Eade and Michael J. Sallnow (London, 1991), 37-50; Eade, 'Order and power at Lourdes'; Coleman, 'From England's Nazareth'; Sallnow, '*Communitas* reconsidered'; Sallnow, 'Pilgrimage and cultural fracture'; Craig, *Wandering Women*, 139-40.

sanctorum limina (this is Turner's liminal phase).[29] Those to be cured might undergo a medical/spiritual crisis and collapse and rise again physically transformed. Their misfortunes reversed, the pilgrims travel home again (Turner's post-liminal phase).

The relevance of Turner's model to miracle stories becomes particularly evident where hagiographers provide additional descriptive detail. Pre-liminality, for example, seems to be expressed in stories in which pilgrims are separated, both voluntarily and involuntarily, from social and familial ties, and from material possessions.[30] Although this is perhaps most forcibly illustrated by judicial penitents excommunicated and exiled from their communities, the pre-liminal is also apparent in stories of illness and disability.[31] There are countless examples of individuals described as unable to function in society in their usual role-defining capacities, such as the musician from Lothian said to have lost his livelihood, and eventually his health, during a time of famine and pestilence. He is described going to St Æbbe's shrine at Coldingham 'weak and naked' (*debilis et nudus*).[32] Other collections

---

[29] *Limina* is frequently the word used for a saint's shrine in miracle collections. There are twenty-three examples in the *Miracula S. Frideswidae*. Prior Philip, 'De miraculis Sanctae Frideswidae', in *Acta Sanctorum*, Octobris, viii, edited by J. Van Kacke et al. (Brussels, 1853), 567-90. The idea of the shrine being a liminal place, 'the joining of heaven and earth', is also prominent in Peter Brown's work, for example, Brown, *Cult*, 1.

[30] As epitomised in the man who, 'leaving his land, home and familiar faces, undertook the labour of pilgrimage' (*terra namque et cognacione et domo relicta, peregrinacionis laborem arripuit*). *Vita et miracula S. Æbbe virginis*, in *The Miracles of St Æbbe of Coldingham and St Margaret of Scotland*, edited and translated by Robert Bartlett, 36.

[31] Judicial penitents were perpetrators of serious crimes whose pilgrimages were imposed by ecclesiastical authorities. In miracle narratives they provide drama and a strong sense of exile due to the fact that they are often described as humbled members of foreign aristocracies, far from home and cultural comforts. For the development of judicial penance, see Jonathan Sumption, *Pilgrimage: An Image of Medieval Religion* (London, 2002), 98-113.

[32] *Miracula S. Æbbe virginis*, 38-41. Men and women 'unable to work' due to illness is a common motif. Examples include *Miracula S. Æbbe virginis*, 56; Reginald of Durham, *Libellus de vita et miraculis S. Godrici, heremitae de Finchale*, edited by Joseph Stevenson, Surtees Society, 20 (London, 1845), 441; Thomas of Monmouth, *The Life and Miracles of St William of Norwich*, edited and translated by Augustus Jessopp and Montague R. James (Cambridge, 1896), 147.

relate stories of cruel abandonment, such as wives deserted by their husbands, a woman thrown out of her house by her stepmother, and a crippled boy neglected by his parents.[33] Some are reduced to begging, living on the margins of society.[34] After being spurned by her family and friends, one blind woman is reportedly forced into mendicancy before her sixteenth birthday.[35] Thus, even before pilgrim protagonists have set out on their journeys, many are already depicted as detached from their usual social and familial networks, becoming what Turner referred to as 'liminal' or, at least, 'liminoid'.[36]

Turner described the liminal phase as a state of transition, 'a time and place of withdrawal', in which initiates passively move – through ordeal, pain and suffering – from the mundane to the sacred.[37] Twelfth-century hagiographers similarly depict pilgrims' journeys in terms of great suffering. Thomas of Monmouth recounts the agonising walk to St William's shrine in Norwich undertaken by a woman whose legs were so crippled and deformed that she was only able to move a finger's length at a time.[38] However, it is at the saint's shrine where the pilgrim's suffering is shown reaching its climax. Dramatic accounts of weeping, wailing, and spontaneous bleeding are not uncommon. Canterbury cathedral is often depicted as the site of such scenes: in the throes of a cure one woman rips away her veil, claws at her clothes and falls to the floor, while another drops to the ground and spends the

---

[33] *Miracula S. Frideswidae*, 574, 586; William of Malmesbury, *Gesta pontificum Anglorum: Volume I. Text and Translation*, edited and translated by Michael Winterbottom with the assistance of Rodney M. Thomson (Oxford, 2007), 648; *Miracula S. Ivonis*, lxix; *The Miracles of the Hand of St James*, translated by Brian Kemp, *Berkshire Archaeological Journal*, 65 (1970), 14-16; *The Book of St Gilbert*, edited and translated by Raymonde Foreville and Gillian Keir (Oxford, 1987), 329-31.

[34] Turner defines marginality as living on the edges, or on the lowest rungs, of structured society. Turner, *Ritual Process*, 128, 125.

[35] *Miracula S. Frideswidae*, 578.

[36] That is, 'quasi-liminal': exhibiting a large percentage of liminal traits. Turner and Turner, *Image and Pilgrimage*, 34-35.

[37] Turner, *Ritual Process*, 167. The liminal 'accept arbitrary punishment without complaint': Turner, *Ritual Process*, 95.

[38] *Life and Miracles of St William of Norwich*, 242-43.

whole day rolling about in convulsions.³⁹ In such cases, individuals rise again, physically transformed and spiritually renewed. Finally, in what we might interpret as the post-liminal phase, pilgrims are shown being incorporated back into society with public ritual celebration such as the ringing of bells, the singing of the *Te Deum*, and the symbolic taking of food.⁴⁰ The recipients of miraculous cures are reunited with their families, and hagiographers frequently emphasise the fact that pilgrims return *ad propria* (literally 'to their own').⁴¹

Turner's rite-of-passage model can be applied to most miracle stories, irrespective of whether or not the miracle beneficiary makes a pilgrimage to a saint's shrine. Healing miracles in particular may be construed as a rite of death and rebirth, a theme made more explicit in cases of miraculous resuscitation.⁴² In an example from William of Canterbury's *Miracula S. Thomae Cantuariensis*, the body of a cancerous girl is shown to be decomposing in front of her family's eyes. William describes how the cancer had eaten into Cecilia's thighs, exposing the bone, and exuding an intolerable stench which keeps her friends away. In line with Turner's liminal phase, the girl is separated from society: her friends desert her and, finally presumed dead, she is carried from the family home and left

---

³⁹ Benedict of Peterborough, *Miracula S. Thomae Cantuariensis*, edited by James C. Robertson, *Materials for the History of Thomas Becket, Archbishop of Canterbury*, volume 2, Rolls Series, 67 (London, 1876), 86, 60.

⁴⁰ One cured pilgrim threw a feast to celebrate with his neighbours and friends. Eadmer of Canterbury, 'Vita Sancti Dunstani archiepiscopi Cantuariensis', in *Lives and Miracles of Saints Oda, Dunstan and Oswald*, edited and translated by Andrew J. Turner and Bernard J. Muir (Oxford, 2006), 162. For other significant examples, see *Book of St Gilbert*, 270, 272-74; *Miracula S. Ivonis*, lxxx.

⁴¹ The phrase is particularly prominent in the Godric and Frideswide collections. *Miraculis S. Godrici*, 392-93, 394, 396, 404, 405, 417, 421, 481; *Miracula S. Frideswidae*, 581, 580, 567, 585.

⁴² On the theme of death and rebirth, see Raymond Van Dam, *Leadership and Community in Late Antique Gaul* (Berkeley and London, 1992), 260-64; Van Gennep, *Rites of Passage*, 159-62. Turner likens liminality to death: Turner, *Ritual Process*, 95. For further comparisons of the two rites, see Frederick S. Paxton, *Christianizing Death: The Creation of a Ritual Process in Early Medieval Europe* (Ithaca and London, 1990).

in an outhouse.⁴³ Moreover, Cecilia is depicted as exhibiting some of the classic Turnerian symptoms of liminality, notably refusing to eat and drink, seeming to be mentally withdrawn and, most telling of all, taking on the appearance of 'one neither dead nor living'.⁴⁴ Her condition is literally one 'betwixt and between' in Turnerian parlance.⁴⁵ Due to the zealous prayers of her father, Cecilia is eventually revived and her body miraculously restored to health. Her reintegration into society is symbolised by another rite of incorporation: the taking of food.⁴⁶

The most significant event in any miracle narrative, of course, is the transition from liminality back to normality, the point at which God restores the world to proper structural order. In healing miracles this is usually a social, as much as a medical, process, as the cure of Cecila's anti-social body nicely demonstrates. As her gaping wound closes, so the breach in the community is sealed as she is welcomed back by friends and family. Collectively, miracle narratives process a whole gamut of non-conforming misfits through a virtual rite of passage and create an idealised, if not slightly homogenised, Christian end-product. From this perspective, we might argue that God and the Christian community are shown collaborating to fashion an ordered, harmonious world on structural-functional principles.

Such a textual adaptation of the rite-of-passage model takes ritual beyond the level of historical reality and into the collective minds of medieval hagiographers. The rite of passage is no longer a pilgrimage undertaken in a literal and historical sense, but a literary contrivance applicable to the entire text. Characters in the narratives are caught up, and carried along, by a rite-of-passage

---

⁴³ A rite-of-passage neophyte may be treated as a corpse: Victor Turner, 'Betwixt and between: the liminal period in Rites de Passage', in *The Forest of Symbols: Aspects of Ndembu Ritual*, edited by Victor Turner (Ithaca and London, 1967), 96.

⁴⁴ Nec mortui speciem nec viventis exhibebat. William of Canterbury, *Miracula S. Thomae Cantuariensis*, edited by James C. Robertson, *Materials for the History of Thomas Becket, Archbishop of Canterbury*, volume 1, Rolls Series, 67 (London, 1876), 191. 'Neither living nor dead from one aspect, and both living and dead from another': Turner, 'Betwixt and between', 97.

⁴⁵ Turner, 'Betwixt and between', 93-111.

⁴⁶ William of Canterbury, *Miracula S. Thomae*, 190-93.

framework and agenda from the moment they step onto the page. Even if not always made explicit, most miracle beneficiaries notionally travel a rite-of-passage narrative journey, simply by undergoing some sort of misfortune and transition.

This type of structural analysis does not, of course, presuppose that medieval writers consciously set out to craft their texts around a pre-existing rite-of-passage blueprint; rather that they unconsciously shaped their narratives around mental structures and story-telling patterns which, arguably, change little over time.[47] However, any attempt to make a rite-of-passage approach to the miracle genre sociological meaningful requires a little more explanation. In order to do this, we must look more deeply at the crux of such an interpretation: ritual. What exactly is ritual, how does it work, and what, if anything, can a ritual approach to miracle narratives reveal about the relationship between hagiographical texts and social reality?

Myth and Ritual: Structure and Function Revisited

The anthropologist Clifford Geertz defined ritual as a cultural performance which attempts to enact, or 'materialise' an imagined world. The result is a fusion of two different realities: the 'world as lived and the world as imagined'.[48] Claude Lévi-Strauss expressed these co-existing components in linguistic terms, placing the 'world as imagined' in the synchronic domain of 'code', and the 'world as lived' in the diachronic dimension of 'message'. 'Code' represented a univocal, abstract, systematic structure, while 'message' comprised variable, constantly evolving units.[49] In this scenario, ritual

---

[47] The idea that 'the human mind is everywhere one and the same' is a frequent proposition of structuralist thinkers, for example Claude Lévi-Strauss, *Myth and Meaning* (London, 1978), 15.

[48] Clifford Geertz, 'Religion as a cultural system', in *The Interpretation of Cultures: Selected Essays*, edited by Clifford Geertz (New York, 1973), 112-22.

[49] Claude Lévi-Strauss, 'The structural study of myth', in *Structural Anthropology*, translated by Claire Jacobson and Brooke G. Schoepf (London, 1963), 206-31. These ideas originated with the linguist Ferdinand de Saussure. See Ferdinand de Saussure, *Premier cours de linguistique générale: d'après les cahiers d'Albert Riedlinger*, edited and translated by George Wolf (Oxford, 1996), 65-66.

mediates between the two, attempting to represent belief (code) in practice (message).

This structural explanation helps towards an understanding of hagiographical writing which, with its tenacious adherence to literary convention and Christian precedent, particularly lends itself to a synchronic reading. Over and above their specific historical details, miracle stories changed very little over a wide range of space and time, but continuously replayed the same structural elements.[50] Although protagonists ostensibly move through a historical, temporal dimension, their slippage towards uniformity and conformity demonstrates that they have, to a greater or lesser extent, been appropriated by a synchronic discourse. Within this stable framework, historical processes are simplified, regulated and subtly reshaped.

Lévi-Strauss was among a group of prominent cultural anthropologists who used the relationship between the synchronic and diachronic to formulate theories concerning an oral narrative form which repeated the same pattern of oppositions and correlations 'over and over again': myth.[51] Myth, in this context, was a 'sacred story', and might be described as the unobtainable 'imagined' world which ritual attempts to re-enact.[52] An important aspect of myth-and-ritual theory is that mythology provides a convincing 'pretence' of historical reality.[53] As far as contemporary audiences were concerned, myths were not mere stories but 'living reality', expressing collective beliefs.[54] However, myths really are

---

[50] As recognized, for example, by Patricia R. Morison, 'The Miraculous and French Society, *c.* 950-1100', unpublished doctoral thesis (University of Oxford, 1983), 70-71.

[51] Lévi-Strauss, *Myth and Meaning*, 34. 'Myth-and-ritual' theories have produced a huge amount of scholarship.

[52] For example, Émile Durkheim, *The Elementary Forms of Religious Life*, translated by Carol Cosman (Oxford, 2001, repr. 2008), 71; Turner, *Ritual Process*, 154.

[53] Roland Barthes, *Mythologies*, translated by Annette Lavers, 2nd edn (London, 1973), 140-55. Barthes thought that 'myth' acts within a 'second-order semiological system' and masquerades as historical truth. Barthes, *Mythologies*, 117-49. Also see Lévi-Strauss, *Myth and Meaning*, 35; Lévi-Strauss, *The Savage Mind*, 2nd edn (London, 1972), 24.

[54] Bronislaw Malinowski, 'Myth in primitive psychology', in *Malinowski and the Work of Myth*, edited by Ivan Strenski (Princeton, 1992), 81.

'lived' through ritual. Ritual brings mythical time into the present by 'projecting' its participants back into the 'mythical epoch'.[55]

Victor Turner likened mythological discourse to hagiography, and miracle stories of twelfth-century England indeed conform to many mythological imperatives, not least in creating exemplary models and disseminating belief.[56] However, perhaps the most significant parallel between miracle stories and myth is that they both combine the synchronic and the diachronic in a characteristically 'duplicitous' way. Like myth, miracle stories allegedly refer to events fixed in time, but simultaneously incorporate other levels of reality.[57] Moreover, miracle stories also provide a good illustration of the complex relationship between myth and ritual. 'Myth' is shown being ritually enacted through pilgrimage in the stories, and transformed back again into narrative 'myth' by hagiography. Hagiographical 'myth' is, in its turn, read to medieval audiences who, we might imagine, are inspired to convert it once more into ritual through devotional acts such as pilgrimage.[58] In this respect, we might even argue that the miracle narrative itself is a form of textual ritual, taking the reader – as much as the protagonist – through a virtual rite of passage.[59]

A 'myth-and-ritual' interpretation of miracle narratives, then, provides insight into the structural mechanics of miracle stories,

---

[55] Mercia Eliade, *The Myth of the Eternal Return*, translated by Willard R. Trask (London, 1955), 34-36. It could be said that three time dimensions are represented in miracle stories: sacred/mythical time, liturgical/ritual time, and profane/chronological time. The first is circular, the second cyclical and the third linear. On the Christianisation of medieval time, see Van Dam, *Leadership*, 277-300.

[56] Turner and Turner, *Image and Pilgrimage*, 23. For this aspect of mythology, see Malinowski, 'Myth', 83.

[57] Lévi-Strauss, *Myth and Meaning*, 36. For 'mythical time' see Lévi-Strauss, 'Structural study of myth', 209-10; Eliade, *Eternal Return*, 20-21.

[58] Indeed, it is known that many hagiographical texts were utilised in this way. For example, the readings of the *passio*, in which the sufferings of the saints were 'publicly re-enacted', have been described by Peter Brown as 'a moment of ritual power'. Brown, *Cult*, 82-84. For another type of ritual engagement with hagiographical texts, see the work of Kathryn Rudy. Kathryn Rudy, 'A guide to mental pilgrimages: Paris, Bibliothèque de l'Arsenal MS. 212', *Zeitschrift für Kunstgeschichte*, 63 (2000), 494-515.

[59] Lévi-Strauss calls myth a 'thought ritual': Lévi-Strauss, *Anthropology and Myth*, translated by Roy Willis (Oxford, 1987), 201.

and possibilities as to their reception. Yet, to make full use of ritual analysis we must also look at one of the mainstays of this type of approach: function. What did social rituals hope to achieve, and what can functional theory tell us about the intended sociological purpose of these hagiographical texts?

The answer can be found by returning to a fundamental Durkheimian idea: that ritual acts as a social-bonding mechanism. That is, in appearing to strengthen the bond between men and God, what ritual is really doing is strengthening the ties between the individual and society.[60] At the most basic level, this explanation suggests that ritual encourages a common sense of belonging, purpose, and corporate identity: 'consensus', 'concord' and 'solidarity' in Peter Brown's late-Roman terminology. However, ritual is also said to come into play especially in times of danger or crisis. When the integrity of a social unit comes under threat, ritual helps the community to confront and dispel its fears: a theory first formulated with respect to death rituals, and extended by Victor Turner to other 'countervailing rites' such as Halloween.[61] Myth-and-ritual theories provide an added strand to the argument. Lévi-Strauss had interpreted myth, with its oppositional determinants, as a problem-solving dialectic.[62] By symbolically simplifying, exaggerating and ultimately negating human fears, myth was 'capable of overcoming (real) contradictions'.[63]

A ritual (or mythical) reading of miracle narratives might then suggest that these medieval stories not only served to inculcate a sense of Christian identification and solidarity, but that they also answered deeper psycho-sociological needs. Miracle stories, like myth, paint a picture of a world which is comfortingly static and

---

[60] Durkheim, *Elementary Forms*, 171.
[61] Bronislaw Malinowski, 'Death and the reintegration of the group', in *Magic, Science and Religion: And Other Essays*, edited by Bronislaw Malinowski (Garden City, New York, 1954), 47-53. Turner, *Ritual Process*, 172-82.
[62] Lévi-Strauss, *Myth and Meaning*, 18-19; Lévi-Strauss, *Savage Mind*, 79-86, 135-60.
[63] Kenelm O. L. Burridge, 'Lévi-Strauss and myth', in *The Structural Study of Myth and Totemism*, edited by Edmund Leach (London, 1967), 99; Lévi-Strauss, *Structural Anthropology*, 229. Also see Lévi-Strauss, *Savage Mind*, 30-33, 130-31.

safe. They re-enact familiar scenarios, and seem to offer mythological solutions to imagined or real problems. On a personal level, this is a credible notion. Protagonists in the narratives are shown encountering a Halloween-like world in which mankind's most basic fears – sickness, disability, disfigurement, poverty and even death – are horrifically magnified, but are nonetheless conquerable. An edifying and comforting fiction is created whereby all oppositional forces are decisively vanquished.[64]

However, a ritual interpretation might also ask whether miracle texts symbolically expressed and resolved underlying fears in a broader social context. Regarding miracle collections as a collective cultural discourse, we might turn to wider themes within western Christianity. The greatest output of English miracle writing fell within a particularly intense period of Christian renewal, diversity and change.[65] Between the late eleventh-century 'Gregorian' reform movements and the Fourth Lateran Council (1215) new, and often challenging, forms of religious ways of life were rapidly emerging. Charismatic preachers and reformers such as Robert of Arbrissel, England's Gilbert of Sempringham, and less savoury characters such as the self-styled crusading preacher, Peter the Hermit and the 'heretic' Henry of Le Mans, offered disciples from diverse social backgrounds a variety of different spiritual opportunities. Mainstream Christianity therefore found itself having to adapt to a new and worrisome era of lay religiosity.[66] Men and women not

---

[64] As such, it may be termed a 'ritual of inclusion and exclusion' as defined by Barbara A. Hanawalt, 'Rituals of inclusion and exclusion: hierarchy and marginalization in medieval London', in *Of Good and Ill Repute: Gender and Social Control in Medieval England*, edited by Barbara A. Hanawalt (Oxford, 1998), 18-34.

[65] In her recent monograph, Rachel Koopmans estimates that, between 1080-1220, at least seventy-five collections of posthumous saints' miracles were produced in England. Rachel Koopmans, *Wonderful to Relate: Miracle Stories and Miracle Collecting in High Medieval England* (Philadelphia, 2011), 2.

[66] André Vauchez describes the 'simple faithful' as rising out of historical obscurity at this time: André Vauchez, *The Laity in the Middle Ages: Religious Practices and Experiences*, translated by Margery J. Schneider (London, 1993), xv, 28, 32.

only channelled their pious energies into pilgrimage, but also into practices which occasionally hovered on the fringes of orthodoxy.[67]

Miracle collections certainly seem to provide evidence for the huge take-up of popular piety in twelfth-century England. However, in promulgating Christian unity and conformity, it is possible that miracle narratives did not just reflect the spiritual energy of the time, but that they were also an institutional response to it.[68] Compared to later centuries, the twelfth has been recognised as a time of relative religious tolerance and freedom of expression.[69] In England, localised heterodox beliefs and practices generally escaped outside censure, and it was not until after the Fourth Lateran Council that ideas about heresy were formalised and an institutional procedure was set up to counter its perceived threat.[70] Before this time, ecclesiastical authorities generally tried to include and modify, rather than suppress and exclude, dissident movements: an attitude Herbert Grundmann calls a 'tactic of incorporation'.[71] From this viewpoint, it could be argued that twelfth-century cults encouraged pilgrimage as part of a localised, or more general, open-arms policy, and that miracle stories 'mythologize' this cultural ideal.

Although ritual approaches to twelfth-century miracle collections are not entirely new, the narratives are often simply regarded as windows through which to view medieval ritual

---

[67] See, for example, Robert I. Moore, 'Heresy, repression and social change in the age of Gregorian reform', in *Christendom and its Discontents: Exclusion, Persecution and Rebellion, 1000-1500*, edited by Scott L. Waugh and Peter D. Diehl (Cambridge, 1996), 19-46; Herbert Grundmann, *Religious Movements in the Middle Ages*, translated by Steven Rowan (London, 1995).

[68] For another institutional response to twelfth-century cultural changes, see Dominique Iogna-Prat, *Order and Exclusion: Cluny and Christendom Face Heresy, Judaism, and Islam (1000-1150)*, translated by Graham Robert Edwards (Ithaca and London, 1998).

[69] Edmund Peters, *Heresy and Authority in Medieval Europe: Documents in Translation* (London, 1980), 165-67.

[70] For 'localism' and heterodox beliefs in England, see Carl S. Watkins, *History and the Supernatural in Medieval England* (Cambridge, 2007), 69-76. For the different reactions to religious dissent and heresy in the twelfth and thirteenth centuries see, for example, Grundmann, *Religious Movements*, 22-23; Jeffrey Richards, *Sex, Dissidence and Damnation: Minority Groups in the Middle Age*, 2nd edn (London and New York, 1994), 9-14.

[71] Grundmann, *Religious Movements*, 18.

practices played out in social reality.[72] However, adapting ritual theories as textual analysis enables us to look at the ritual function of the text, rather than at the ritual function of medieval pilgrimage. Unlike the work of Victor Turner, that of myth-and-ritual theorists do not seem to have been taken up by medievalists. Nonetheless, in bridging the awkward gap between conceptual forms and lived reality, myth-and-ritual theories offer a different perspective on the relationship between society and culture, and allow us not so much to disentangle the troublesome mixture of fact and fiction in miracle narratives, as to read these two levels of reality as mutually dependent components whose fusion helped medieval people make sense of their world.

Structuralism Revisited

The aim of this chapter has been to give a brief demonstration of some of the ways in which social and cultural anthropology has influenced miracle scholarship over the past thirty years, and to suggest how some of anthropology's most popular theories, such as structural-functionalism and ritual theory, might be re-deployed as a type of textual analysis to offer fresh ways of thinking about miracle narratives.

Peter Brown, Victor Turner and 'myth-and-ritual' scholars were all structuralist theorists, framing their ideas in terms of generic social models. Structuralism is a form of cultural anthropology concerned with thought structures, or, more precisely, with mental models employed by humans to make their world more intelligible. An important element of structuralism is that it offers a synchronic viewpoint: in its 'quest for the invariant' it privileges continuity, and regularity, over change and diversity.[73] In reducing the chaos of reality to ordered patterns, structuralism is also often used to resolve the juxtapositions of its own creation which may, or may not, also exist in the real world. Peter Brown is perhaps the best

---

[72] As seen in Robert I. Moore, 'Between sanctity and superstition: saints and their miracles in the age of revolution', in *The Work of Jacques Le Goff and the Challenges of Medieval History*, edited by Miri Rubin (Woodbridge, 1997), 57-58; Yarrow, *Saints and their Communities*, 18-19.

[73] Lévi-Strauss, *Myth and Meaning*, 6.

known importer of the structural method into the study of medieval cults, explaining saint devotion in terms of a conceptual domain, where the contrary categories of heaven and earth, the living and the dead, and the public and private met and coalesced.[74] Brown explained how, at the shrine of the saint, these symbolic polarities resolved their structural oppositions, creating what Victor Turner called '*communitas*', and what Lévi-Strauss defined as 'myth'.

Structural and ritual approaches, such as those of Turner and Lévi-Strauss, are not without their detractors who argue that such modes of analysis are essentialist, reductionist and a-historical in nature, and carry with them the risk of imposing modern concepts anachronistically onto medieval culture.[75] To a certain extent these critics are correct: 'aiming at the discovery of general laws', structuralism does indeed ignore historical specificity and sets up abstract models to which, inevitably, not every element will perfectly conform.[76] For this reason, structural anthropology is often seen as antithetical to historical enquiry: social models, it is said, place historians at some mental distance from the concrete realities of the tangible, factual world.[77] The Turners' application of ritual theory to pilgrimage is particularly contested, and not even

---

[74] Brown, *Cult*, 1-22.

[75] See, for example, Buc, *Dangers of Ritual*, 1-4, and passim. Turner's ritual theories are critiqued in Eade and Sallnow's anthology of essays, *Contesting the Sacred*. Also see Coleman, 'Do you Believe in Pilgrimage?', and Michael J. Sallnow, '*Communitas* Reconsidered'.

[76] Alfred R. Radcliffe-Brown, 'The methods of ethnology and social anthropology', in *Method in Social Anthropology: Selected Essays by A. R. Radcliffe-Brown*, edited by Mysore N. Srinivas (London, 1958), 25. A 'model' may be defined as 'an intellectual construct which simplifies reality in order to emphasize the recurrent, the constant and the typical, which it presents in the form of clusters or traits or attributes'. Peter Burke, *Sociology and History* (London, 1980), 35.

[77] Burke, *Sociology*, 35-37; Bob Scribner, 'Historical anthropology of Early Modern Europe', in *Problems in the Historical Anthropology of Early Modern Europe*, edited by R. Po-Chia Hsia and Robert W. Scribner (Wiesbaden, 1997), 15; Bernard S. Cohn, 'History and anthropology: the state of play', in *An Anthropologist Among the Historians and Other Essays* (Oxford, 1990), 19-21; Simon Coleman and John Elsner, *Pilgrimage: Past and Present: Sacred Travel and Sacred Space in the World Religions* (London, 1995), 198-200. For comparisons of the historical and anthropological methods, see Cohn, *An Anthropologist*, 1-47; Lévi-Strauss, 'History and anthropology', 1-27.

Peter Brown escapes similar types of scholarly censure.[78] In short, postmodern scholarship, which privileges notions of diversity and specificity, does appear less than comfortable with framing history in terms of universal mentalities.

Although it is true that structural interpretations of miracle narratives cannot accurately reconstruct the medieval past, it does not necessarily follow that these methods are unworkable in a historical context *per se*. Structural anthropology is not, as some historians assert, a cognitive device which was alien to the middle ages. On the contrary, twelfth-century writers were structural thinkers thinking in terms of a structural world. Not only did the intellectual culture of the time seek to order ideas and experiences in increasingly standard and formalised ways, but the emphasis on structure and slow-change was particularly pertinent at a time when the Church aspired towards regularity, stability and conformity in the face of rapidly encroaching social and religious changes. Unlike the postmodern world, diversity and individuality – particularly in a Christian context – were seen as negative, and as potentially dangerous, forces. Faced with this challenging new world, twelfth-century religious writers must often have found the mythological 'quest for the invariant' particularly desirable.[79]

Miracle stories, moreover, are particularly suited to structural analysis. The criticisms of reductionism and a-historicism are less

---

[78] Anthropological volumes compiled as critiques of Turner's pilgrimage paradigm include: Eade and Sallnow's *Contesting the Sacred*; Coleman and Eade's *Reframing Pilgrimage* and Alan Morinis, *Sacred Journeys: The Anthropology of Pilgrimage* (London, 1992). Studies which are specifically medieval in context include Nicholas Vincent, 'The pilgrimage of the Angevin kings of England 1154-1272', in *Pilgrimage: The English Experience from Becket to Bunyan*, edited by Colin Morris and Peter Roberts (Cambridge, 2002), 12-45; Caroline Walker Bynum, 'Women's stories, women's symbols: a critique of Victor Turner's theory of liminality', in *Fragmentation and Redemption: Essays on Gender and the Human Body in Medieval Religion* (London, 2002), 27-51. Other anthropological deconstructionists are discussed and listed in Coleman, 'Do you believe in pilgrimage?', 356-57. For a critique of Peter Brown, see Paul Antony Hayward, 'Demystifying the role of sanctity in western Christendom', in *The Cult of Saints in Late Antiquity and the Early Middle Ages: Essays on the Contribution of Peter Brown*, edited by John Howard-Johnston and Paul Antony Hayward (Oxford, 1999), 115-42.

[79] Lévi-Strauss, *Myth and Meaning*, 6.

relevant for a genre which, in so strictly adhering to literary and Christian precedents, produces narratives which intrinsically changed little over the centuries. Miracle stories mediate between reassuring timeless tradition on the one hand, and the caprices of real life on the other. They are comfortingly static, combining and re-combining the same familiar elements, and providing reassurance that the past is always present.

Structural anthropology, then, serves to remind us that miracle accounts are not always transparent windows into the medieval world, and that *dramatis personae* of the stories are as much products of a shared cultural mentality as they are of their individual historical circumstance. A structural-functionalist reading of miracle narratives, we might argue, delves into a community's collective psychology. It helps illuminate society's aspirations and fears, and suggests one way in which religious authorities may have responded to life's uncertainties: through story-telling. Furthermore, examining miracle stories through a 'structural' lens not only provides an alternative way to think about the function of these texts, but it also helps in untangling the relationship between fact and fiction highlighted in the quotation at the beginning of the chapter. In particular, it reveals miracle narratives in a new light: as a reassuring compromise between reality and ideology packaged in a simple, but psychologically satisfying, way.

Structuralism also has a possible further application. It might be used to reflect upon how we, as historians, unconsciously structure and shape our own understanding of the past. Historians, like hagiographers, structure their stories around culturally-accepted narrative frameworks. Their thought patterns are influenced by those around them, and by those who have gone before. In this respect, a collection of essays showcasing new approaches to miracles in the medieval West is particularly welcome. It is a much-needed reminder of the importance of continually re-framing, and re-assessing, our interpretations of the medieval world: interpretations which, after all, represent our own unconscious compromises between fact and fiction.

MIRACLES, BELIEF AND CHRISTIAN MATERIALITY: RELIC'ING IN TWELFTH-CENTURY MIRACLE NARRATIVES

Simon Yarrow

There is no kind of report that rises so easily, and spreads so quickly especially in the country places and provincial towns, as those concerning marriages, insomuch that the two young persons of equal condition never see each other twice, but the whole neighbourhood immediately join them together ... do not the same passions, and others still stronger, incline the generality of mankind to believe and report, with the greatest vehemence and assurance, all religious miracles?[1]

In his Haskell lectures of 1978, Peter Brown drew attention to the lingering presence among the 'mental furniture' of historians, of Hume's elitist, two-tier perspective on 'the religious mind', and introduced functionalism as a way of avoiding its distorting effects on history.[2] The theme of 'elite and popular religion' has continued to exercise historians, the *Ecclesiastical History Society* revisiting it as recently as 2006. Contributions to the proceeding volume of *Studies in Church History*, and to its preceding volume on *Signs, Wonders and Miracles*, confirmed the enduring afterlife of the two-tier tradition.[3] Some contributors were still quite happy to work within it, and no obvious alternative approach emerged from

---

[1] David Hume, *An Enquiry Concerning Human Understanding: A Critical Edition*, edited by Tom L. Beauchamp (Oxford, 2000), 89.
[2] Peter Brown, *The Cult of the Saints: Its Rise and Function in Latin Christianity* (Chicago, 1981), 13.
[3] *Signs, Wonders, Miracles: Representations of Divine Power in the Life of the Church*, edited by Kate Cooper and Jeremy Gregory, Studies in Church History, 41 (Woodbridge, 2005).

them.[4] This has in part been due to the narrowing confidence among historians during the 1990s in the possibility of retrieving unmediated popular religious belief from the sources, a development we shall explore below. But it is also arguably a consequence of the social template the sources themselves use broadly to characterise lived religion. Witness the comments of Guibert of Nogent (d. 1124) on the suspect cult of a 'common boy, the squire of a certain knight', on an estate near Beauvais:

> After some peasants, desirous of novelty, began to honour him, suddenly all the nearby ignorant country folk carried oblations and candles to his grave ... feigned cases of deafness, pretended bouts of madness ... we have heard how such things are bandied about in repeated whispers, and we have witnessed ridiculous deeds performed during the translation of relics ... what can I say about others [i.e. saints] whom commoners – envious of these saints just mentioned [Saints Martin and Rémy] – create every day in every village and in every town.[5]

Into these equally dismissive descriptions of popular religious practice, separated by over half a millennium, are written two distinct conceptions of authority in matters of religious belief in miracles: in Hume's case a philosophical argument; in the case of Guibert, a doctrinal and pastoral argument. Hume's understanding of miracles existed on metaphysical and empirical levels. His well-known statement, 'a miracle is a violation of the laws of nature',[6] is a version of Thomas Aquinas's definition of miracles as events

---

[4] A series of recently published lectures given by Caroline Walker Bynum entitled *Christian Materiality: An Essay on Religion in Late Medieval Europe* (New York, 2011), reflects on this binary in the context of object-oriented religion; see 129-31, and particularly note 14.

[5] 'Cumque id rustici rerum novarum cupidi celebrassent, repente oblationes et cerei ab omni agrestium pagensium vicinia ad ejus tumulum comportantur ... fictitiae surditates, affectatae vesaniae ... Crebro teri perspicimus ista susurro, et facta feretrorum circumlatione ridicula ... quid de eis proferam, quos praefatorum aemulum per villas ac oppida quotidie vulgus creat?'. Guibert of Nogent, *'Monodies' and 'On the Relics of Saints': The Autobiography and a Manifesto of a French Monk from the Time of the Crusades*, translated by Joseph McAlhany and Jay Rubenstein (London, 2011), 206-07; and Guibert of Nogent, '*De sanctis et eorum pigneribus*', edited by Robert B. C. Huygens, Corpus Christianorum, 127 (Turnhout, 1993), 79-175.

[6] Hume, *An Enquiry Concerning Human Understanding*, 86.

contra naturam.[7] Hume's proof for miracles rested on the survival of probability from the mutual destruction of reported sense perceptions of a supposed miracle event. That is, the weighing of rival testimonies according to reliability, determined levels of probability of a miracle having taken place. Since Hume regarded it as impossible to perceive anything in nature that did not conform to nature's laws, it followed that the proof of a miracle depended upon such testimony as the falsehood of which required a miracle itself to corroborate. In other words, Hume's position did not rule out miracles but deferred their confirmation to an infinite regression of ultimately improbable testimonies to such, he claimed, as even the most trustworthy of human beings were limited, but which, he opined, were typically found circulating among country-folk and provincial types.

Of course, Hume's empiricist argument against crediting the senses with that which cannot be sensed was not strictly an argument against crediting God with the ability occasionally to allow us to sense it. Many of Hume's peers, among them Newtonian scientists, were quite happy with this loophole.[8] In this respect they were not as far removed as we think from medieval scholasticism, and monastic learning, as exemplified by Guibert of Nogent. The alternative to Hume's impossible criteria produced two related problems: how does one know when God has intervened (a question of the scrutiny and regulation of evidence), and secondly, what does one do with the miraculous wheat having once winnowed away the chaff (a question of interpretation)? Before considering Guibert of Nogent's twelfth-century critique of the cult of saints' relics it would be useful to adduce some evidence for the intellectual inheritance that shaped his thinking on these questions of scrutiny and interpretation.

---

[7] Benedicta Ward, *Miracles and the Medieval Mind: Theory, Record and Event, 1000-1215*, 2nd edn (Aldershot, 1987), 3-9.

[8] See Charles S. Peirce, *Collected Papers*, edited by Charles Hartshorne and Paul Weiss, volume 6, Scientific Metaphysics (Cambridge, Massachusetts, 1935), chapter 5. Also see Jane Shaw, *Miracles in Enlightenment England* (Yale, 2006), 172, who identifies those Newtonian scientists of the mid-eighteenth century who accepted that evidence might periodically demonstrate God's ongoing intervention in his Creation.

Augustine of Hippo had elegant answers to these problems that influenced how the medieval church subsequently learned to detect and explain when the relics in their safekeeping worked miracles. Since miracles were signs of heavenly grace revealed directly to the faithful they were a form of authority to which the faithful could appeal that bypassed other divinely ordained institutions such as the state or the church. Though anyone in theory could petition a saint in the hope of a miracle, Augustine struck a balance between local innovation and central regulation by insisting on the duty of the clergy to authenticate the miracle experiences of the faithful through their scrutiny and commemoration in written record. Such records, or *libelli miraculorum*, were to be kept at every local shrine. Since Augustine regarded the whole of Creation as a miracle, those events customarily recognized as miracles were not 'against nature' but rather extensions of human perception and intended by God as aids to faith. Miracles were meant for potential converts, for catechumens and for 'slow learners', and so fitted the clergy's task of recording them with a pastoral obligation. Miracle stories were thus concerned not just with the authentication of miracles but with their interpretation as signs of religious values, goals and insights beyond their historical particularity. For this reason they were often associated with preaching and conversion in early hagiographical genres. The theme of hagiography as a vehicle for the 'rehearsal of Christian content',[9] or as 'adjuncts to evangelization'[10] is at the heart of the work of Gregory the Great and Bede, the latter, of course, arguably the chief influence on the twelfth-century English chroniclers and hagiographers whom we shall consider in the rest of this chapter.[11]

---

[9] Kate Cooper, 'Ventriloquism and the miraculous: conversion, preaching, and the martyr *exemplum* in late Antiquity', in *Signs, Wonders, Miracles: Representations of Divine Power in the Life of the Church*, edited by Kate Cooper and Jeremy Gregory, Studies in Church History, 41 (Woodbridge, 2005), 34.

[10] William McCready, *Signs of Sanctity: Miracles in the Thought of Gregory the Great* (Toronto, 1989), 35.

[11] Bertram Colgrave, 'Bede's miracle stories' in *Bede, His Life, Times and Writings*, edited by Alexander Hamilton Thompson (New York, 1966), 222-26; and Benedicta Ward, 'Miracles and history: Bede's miracle stories', in *Famulus Christi: Essays in Commemoration of the Thirteenth Centenary of the Birth of the Venerable Bede*, edited by Gerald Bonner (London, 1976), 72-73.

Guibert of Nogent's treatise on the cult of saints' relics, *De pignoribus sanctorum*, is a combination of biblical interpretation, doctrine and anecdote reflecting on the temptations and abuses associated in his day with these broadly Augustinian arrangements for the monitoring of shrine-centred miracles. It was written *circa* 1120 and provides an invaluable exposé of the more dubious workings of popular relic cults for which churchmen of the early thirteenth century were attempting to establish a legal foundation for regulation in the form of papal canonization.[12]

Guibert counted the veneration of saints and their bodies among those Christian practices held but not formally taught within the faith. The faithful were free to observe these practices provided they did not conflict with the core teachings of the church. Guibert repeatedly berated those bishops and abbots in his north-eastern corner of France who failed to give proper leadership in this matter, and worse, who lent their weight to what he felt were crude money-making scams, a notorious concrete example of which was the cult of the tooth of Christ at St Médard, Soissons, which infuriated him for making a mockery of the Resurrection. Guibert's remedy for this abuse was twofold. Churchmen should stop plundering saints' tombs and circulating their remains, and hagiography should observe more stringent standards of verification. The authenticity of saints' relics was to be properly scrutinized, with reference to venerable tradition (*vetustatis traditio*), or by true writings (*scriptorium veracium*), not by mere opinion (*non opinio*). Guibert mentions turning down requests to write biographies for relics about which nothing was known.

But *scriptorium veracium* did not solely involve demonstrating chains of reliable testimony verifying a saint's relic. For Guibert proper style was a necessary (although not sufficient) aspect of hagiographical composition. Without it, hagiography could obscure true sanctity. He describes some existing biographies as 'writings worse than doggerel, unfit for the ears of swineherds'.[13]

---

[12] André Vauchez, *Sainthood in the Later Middle Ages*, translated by Jean Birrell, 2nd ed (Cambridge, 2005), 22-32.

[13] Porro sunt quaedam de aliquibus scripta, quae multo deteriora neniis ne subulcorum quidem essent auribus inferenda. Guibert of Nogent, '*De sanctis et eorum pigneribus*', 102; Guibert of Nogent, '*Monodies' and 'On the Relics of Saints'*, translated by McAlhany and Rubenstein, 210.

He mentions elsewhere, 'even those that are true are often told in such a ragged and pedestrian style ... that by their awkwardness they defame the saints, and even the least little thing about them seems false'.[14]

Whilst he followed the implication in the title to Gregory of Tours' *Life of the Fathers*, Guibert implied elsewhere that the overuse of the topos, the hagiographer's tool for referencing the ideal of sanctity upon which all saints converged, is a symptom of bad style that carries damaging consequences, 'there are to be sure many stories about all of the saints that serve less to commend their reputation than to defame it among unbelievers'.[15]

False Relics and Good Intentions

The danger to which Guibert alerted churchmen involved in the custodianship of relics is illustrated in twelfth-century English miracle narratives of religious who took liberties in the handling of relics. Gundulf, Bishop of Rochester in the early years of Henry I's reign, was considered such a pious and blameless man that saints allowed him to handle their relics.[16] But other religious were less favoured when they attempted to handle relics for various different purposes. An audacious priest who intervened at the shrine of St Aethelthryth of Ely with three fellow priests, poked a stick into the tomb in order to hook some of the garment inside it, only for it to be snatched back inside by the saint. Those who took part all suffered illness, their leader and his family dying soon after of the plague. The lesson was made clear: 'let any unworthy handlers of relics learn from this that they ought only to dare such a thing with

---

[14] Ubi enim etiam quae vera sunt adeo pannoso, et pedestri, et, ut poetico verbo utar, humi serpenti eloquio proferuntur, imo inconditissime delatrantur, ut cum minime sint, falsissima esse credantur. Guibert of Nogent, '*De sanctis et eorum pigneribus*', 87; Guibert of Nogent, '*Monodies*' *and* '*On the Relics of Saints*', translated by McAlhany and Rubenstein, 195.

[15] Sunt enim quam plurimae super quibusque sanctis relationes, quibus potius eorum praeconium apud infideles impiari poterat. Guibert of Nogent, '*De sanctis et eorum pigneribus*', 87; Guibert of Nogent, '*Monodies*' *and* '*On the Relics of Saints*', translated by McAlhany and Rubenstein, 195.

[16] *The Life of Gundulf, Bishop of Rochester*, edited by Rodney M. Thomson (Toronto, 1977), 53.

purity and humility of heart'.[17] In Goscelin's *Life of Edith*, a monk of Glastonbury attempted to cut fabric away from her shroud and a nun tried to cut away some of her headband. The nun was no doubt appropriately abashed when the dead saint turned her head in stern rebuke of the 'presumptuous woman'.[18] Two monks at Bury St Edmunds, Herman and Tolinus, handled and inspected the saint's relics, Herman even holding an impromptu exhibition of his vest (*camisia*), for which they were punished.[19] With these scare stories in mind the carefully worded statements of humility and awe by hagiographers in the prefaces to their works should not simply be seen as literary filler.

Moreover, Guibert appears to have unsettled many of his readers into asking him for clarification on whether false or misidentified relics might have deleterious effects on those who innocently venerate them. In the former case he assures his readers that, 'anyone who invokes God uncertainly annoys him, but if he faithfully beseeches the one whom he believes to be a saint but who is not a saint, then he still appeases God'.[20] A marginal addition to the only surviving manuscript offers further reassurance on the subject of misidentified relics, creatively citing John 17:22, 'For the Lord said about the saints, "Let them be one, even as we are one"'.[21]

Yet all this runs counter to an abiding theme in the text, that 'who except an utter madman would call for help from somebody

---

[17] Habeant ex hoc quilibet sacrarum indigni attrectatores reliquiarum quia nisi cum cordis munditia et humilitate id debent presumere. *Goscelin of Saint-Bertin: The Hagiography of the Female Saints of Ely*, edited and translated by Rosalind Love (Oxford, 2004), 129.

[18] *Writing the Wilton Women: Goscelin's Legend of Edith and Liber Confortatorius*, edited by Stephanie Hollis (Turnhout, 2005), 72.

[19] *Memorials of St Edmund's Abbey*, edited by Thomas Arnold, volume 1, Rolls Series, 96 (London, 1890), 173-75.

[20] Qui eum de quo est incertus exposcit, irritat, ita eum, si fideliter sanctum illum credens quo non est sanctus exoret, placat. Guibert of Nogent, '*De sanctis et eorum pigneribus*', 108; Guibert of Nogent, '*Monodies*' and '*On the Relics of Saints*', translated by McAlhany and Rubenstein, 216.

[21] Cum enim de eis dominus dicat: ut sit inquit, unum sicut et nos unum sumus. Guibert of Nogent, '*De sanctis et eorum pigneribus*', 108; Guibert of Nogent, '*Monodies*' and '*On the Relics of Saints*', translated by McAlhany and Rubenstein, 216.

about whom there survives not even a lingering hint as to what sort of person he was?'²² The importance of the authenticity of the relic is the basis for Guibert's worry that 'any people might find homes within the sacred precincts behind altars as if upon the highest thrones of the heavenly court, when their history, their birth and life, their days and the character of their death survives in the memory of no living person'.²³ The additional afterthought ignores relics and focuses on the intentionality of the faithful, implying that the channels relics open between God and a petitioner are incidental to the communion of faithful conviction with heavenly grace.

Belief in Objects and Belief in Doctrines

Guibert's work is an invaluable Cook's tour of the whole business of cult promotion and relic veneration in the twelfth century. Guibert sought firm grounds on which to base belief in the miraculous power of relics, working in Augustinian tracks of regulation and pastoral duty. But it seems by the logical implication of his marginal addendum that even (and perhaps especially) the religious walked on unsteady ground when it came to relic-oriented, as distinct from text-oriented, religious practice. Did sincere devotion to false relics frustrate one's efforts at good works? Did the handling of true relics by the unworthy really carry with it danger to life and limb? And in what circumstances did the circulation of relics avoid sliding into the degraded appearance of a financial transaction? Ambiguity accompanied the motivations of those who bought relics, like the nuns of Wilton who paid a staggering 2000s for the relics carried by an itinerant group of

---

[22] De quibus ergo ne suspitio quales fuerint residua quidem extat, qui hos nisi extreme demens, ad pro se interpellandum provocat'. Guibert of Nogent, '*De sanctis et eorum pigneribus*, 100; Guibert of Nogent, '*Monodies' and 'On the Relics of Saints*', translated by McAlhany and Rubenstein, 208.

[23] Illud dicere audebo profanum, quod ararum pone sacraria altissimos tribunalium instar thronos obtinent, quorum tempus, natalis, ac vita, dies quoque et qualitas mortium in nullius viventis memoria resident. Guibert of Nogent, '*De sanctis et eorum pigneribus*', 100; Guibert of Nogent, '*Monodies' and 'On the Relics of Saints*', translated by McAlhany and Rubenstein, 89, 197.

Pictish monks,[24] and Guibert's talk of bishops 'seduced by piles of pilgrim gifts', of a 'marketing-man' (*prolocutor*), calling on him for the casual endorsement of a relic, and the shameful double-dealing of bishops buying and selling the relics of a peasant mistaken for his namesake, St Exuperius.[25] In this uncertain area at any moment spirituality might alarmingly come to resemble commerce and corruption, and for those involved, 'what' in Guibert's words 'would be beneficial for their souls' salvation' could end up being 'turned into shit for their purses'.[26]

It may be that Guibert's precocious reforming sensibilities, as they did in other ecclesiastical matters, placed him alone and uncomfortably ahead of his time, and that many of his contemporaries were willing to turn a blind eye and accept as 'pious invention' what Guibert naively and perhaps, at times, uncharitably attributed to venality.[27] For whatever reason, his treatise cut across the rhetorical plane of contemporary hagiography with criticisms to which historians have sometimes paid the compliment of misidentifying as rational,[28] but which, I would suggest, actually bring us back to and, in comparison with Hume's empirical insight, fruitfully complicate our historical understanding of belief and the two-tier model of religion.

Two-Tiers Revisited

Until now I have shelved discussion of the possibility for historians of recovering popular religious belief in relics from the sources.

---

[24] *Writing the Wilton Women*, 74-75.

[25] Munerum comportatorum blandiente frequentia. Guibert of Nogent, '*De sanctis et eorum pigneribus*', 97; Guibert of Nogent, '*Monodies*' *and* '*On the Relics of Saints*', translated by McAlhany and Rubenstein, 205, 206 and 212.

[26] Si saperent, suarum conducibile saluti animarum, hoc excrementa efficiant crumenarum. Guibert of Nogent, '*De sanctis et eorum pigneribus*', 104; Guibert of Nogent, '*Monodies*' *and* '*On the Relics of Saints*', translated by McAlhany and Rubenstein, 213.

[27] Robert I. Moore, 'Guibert of Nogent and his world', in *Studies in Medieval History Presented to R. H. C. Davis*, edited by Henry Mayr-Harting and Robert I. Moore (London, 1985), 107-18.

[28] Useful discussion of this can be found in John F. Benton, *Self and Society in Medieval France: The Memoirs of Abbot Guibert of Nogent* (Toronto, 1970), 1-31.

Instead I have concentrated on the elite, literate tier and noted the phenomenon of ecclesiastical ambivalence in its interpretations of relic-oriented belief in miracles. I have done so because it is my suspicion that the mental furniture Brown attributes to Hume is a minor variant of what already exists in twelfth-century hagiography, and can be traced back to the Church Fathers and beyond. The Bible itself was equivocal on the subject. Two passages in John's Gospel, 'Jesus did the first of his miracles in Canaan, Galilee, and revealed his glory; and his disciples believed in him' and 'Jesus said to him, unless you see signs and wonders you believe not'[29] must have strengthened Augustine's conviction that miracles were a means to, but a poor goal of, faith.

My hesitation to make claims on behalf of popular religion is that I suspect the resilience of two-tier thinking lies in the willingness, for different reasons, of the literate of all ages to treat object-oriented belief as a rhetorical cover for various forms of strategic and tactical condescension and reduction. Those who would ignore ecclesiastical ambivalence as an authorising technique tend to have firm notions of the church as an arbiter of official religion and would emphasise the literal and prescriptive over the diagnostic matter in Guibert's treatise. More modern reflective confessional and top-down historians of the church have grappled with the apparently rational and credulous character of hagiographers and their sources, seeking to rescue them from the effects of Hume and Guibert's critical pincer movement. This has frequently resulted in special pleading on behalf of important figures like Bede,[30] Gregory the Great,[31] and William of Malmesbury,[32] as at once being above this nonsense and so still reliable for modern historical purposes, but at the same time tolerant of its dissemination, not disingenuously but in good faith for purely didactic purposes for audiences (lay and/or religious depending on how elitist one wants to be) incapable of perceiving

---

[29] *Biblia Sacra Vulgata*, John 2:11; John 4:48.
[30] See Ward, 'Miracles and history', 72-73.
[31] McCready, *Signs of Sanctity*, 111-53.
[32] Rodney M. Thomson, *William of Malmesbury*, 2nd ed (Woodbridge, 2003), 11-38, especially at 22, for discussion of this matter in the work of the twelfth century's most consummate historian-hagiographer.

beyond its surface.[33] For non-confessional social historians the temptation has been to overlook ecclesiastical ambivalence and politely to assume faith as normative then, through an adoption of the view from Hume's armchair, to strip away the social detail (Hume's 'marriage gossip') from belief and qualify the latter as a confused perception of natural causation characteristic of the medieval mind. The trouble with this normative reading of object-oriented belief is that if it does not actually blind us to the clear presence of doubt, uncertainty and perhaps even Humean empiricist concern among medieval folk, then it makes it difficult for us to acknowledge, differentiate and explain it.[34] Peter Brown's functionalist approach, with which I began this chapter, brought compelling social texture to the two-tier model it exposed, but in the process smoothed over the kinds of difference, conflict and anxiety that the rhetorical traces of ambivalence, most dramatically expressed in Guibert's treatise, can sometimes betray, even as they attempt to do otherwise. The implications of the 'fantasies of consensus' most representative of the genre, that Guibert's work approaches from a usefully oblique angle, is interestingly explored in Anne E. Bailey's chapter on the functionalism of textual representations in the present volume.

In short, two-tier religious history risks reproducing the rhetorical grain of the sources, and by doing so commits to blanket assumptions about belief that do not necessarily exist but toward which the sources persuasively work.[35] It might be useful, therefore, to suspend our claims about popular religious belief altogether, and to work, first, from the notion that all medieval people, religious and lay, literate and illiterate, high and low status, were capable of ambivalence when it came to faith, and secondly, to consider the likelihood that relic-oriented religion afforded layers of interpretive and evaluative opportunity to far more diffuse communities than

[33] Steven Justice, 'Did the middle ages believe in their miracles?', *Representations*, 103 (2008), 5-6.
[34] A subject on which Susan Reynolds presciently wrote in Susan Reynolds, 'Social mentalities and the case of medieval scepticism', *Transactions of the Royal Historical Society*, sixth series, 1 (1991), 21-41.
[35] This issue is discussed all the more usefully for its application in a different context by Tom McCaskie, *State and Society and Pre-Colonial Asante* (Cambridge, 1995), 19-23.

text-producing communities might have wished, hence the anxious calls of highly literate reformers like Guibert of Nogent for greater textual regulation and the reduced circulation of relics. Finally, with these two points in mind, I shall sketch an approach that might enable us to trace links, nodes and flows between and through text and object-oriented practices better to reconstruct religious belief in terms of Christian materiality.[36]

Reading Texts for Objects

If we dispense with 'popular religion' then how do we get at those diffuse object-oriented interpretative acts that constitute religion in our sources? Since the linguistic turn, there have been more and less optimistic answers to this question grouped around various discursive approaches to the subject. Carl Watkins has pithily described miracles in twelfth-century English chronicles as 'treacherous'. After judiciously reviewing literary approaches pioneered by, among others, Gabrielle Spiegel and Monica Otter in the 1990s, he has cautioned against their excessively varied readings and apparent abandonment of historical reality.[37] His advocacy of an examination of the degree to which 'audiences are a control on historical representation', represents a pragmatic but arguably insufficiently rigorous response to their interpretive apparatus, but is nevertheless a sensible and safe haven for historians committed to relating texts to 'real' referents.[38] Marcus Bull traces the oscillation of interpretive opportunities between scribes and miracle participants in his study of the twelfth-century miracles of Our

---

[36] My ideas have benefitted from the work of David Graeber, *Toward an Anthropological Theory of Value: The False Coin of Our Own Dreams* (London, 2001), 33-34, 104-106 and, more recently, by the publication of Caroline Walker Bynum's *Christian Materiality*.

[37] Carl S. Watkins, *History and the Supernatural in Medieval England* (Cambridge, 2007), 17.

[38] Michael E. Goodich, '*Mirabilis Deus in sanctis suis*: social history and medieval miracles', in *Signs, Wonders, Miracles: Representations of Divine Power in the Life of the Church*, edited by Kate Cooper and Jeremy Gregory, Studies in Church History, 41 (Woodbridge, 2005), 135-56 and Simon Yarrow, *Saints and their Communities: Miracle Stories in Twelfth-Century England* (Oxford, 2006), 215.

Lady of Rocamadour.[39] His premise that miracles were a common cultural reference point opens miracle stories up to narratological examination, in order to trace processes of attestation into and through texts. Rachel Koopman's recent examination of the socially diffuse authorising processes found in twelfth-century miracle collections, independently corroborates Bull's approach to the dynamics of story-telling but tantalisingly concludes that ultimately, 'so much eludes us'.[40]

So where does this leave us? Miracle narratives belonged to a fixed and self-referencing literary genre. At the same time they claimed and asserted attested routes into real events. The social dynamics they contained, more mundane and diffuse than in any other kind of medieval source, cry out for historical treatment. And yet these are difficult to reconstruct, compressed and encapsulated as they are in narratives rarely susceptible to normal techniques of historical verification by independent sources, and which combine probative with rhetorical techniques including chains and hierarchies of testimony, empirical demonstration, literary topoi, and descriptions of objects being circulated and viewed. We might wish to read these sources not as trading in belief, but as trying to hold many fragments and threads together in arguments for belief, and not just any old belief, but a prescribed version of belief, in the face of potential uncertainty and conflict that cuts across and erases the popular-elite divide. But this is not an argument for endless inter-textual readings of sources, nor for the convergence of all religious practices ultimately on texts. Historians must attempt to relate their sources to real people.[41]

Miracle narratives were compressed meditations on doubt that piled on rhetorical pressure so that their audiences might absorb prescribed beliefs. It is entirely likely that people absorbed these arguments for belief in different contexts for different reasons, and

---

[39] *The Miracles of Our Lady of Rocamadour: Analysis and Translation*, edited and translated by Marcus Bull (Woodbridge, 1999), 11.

[40] Rachel Koopmans, *Wonderful to Relate Miracle Stories and Miracle Collecting in High Medieval England* (Philadelphia, 2011), 21.

[41] In this I wholly concur with Janet L. Nelson's citation of Marc Bloch in her 'Monks, secular men and masculinity, *c.* 900', in *Masculinity in Medieval Europe*, edited by Dawn M. Hadley (London, 1999), 138.

that through their own interpretive and evaluative efforts, and embodied experiences before audiences gathered at shrines, they might have aspired to influence receptions of these beliefs among subsequent audiences. In which case we might usefully read our sources as feeding into and out of a rich and many-layered experience of Christian material practice. In our attempts to do so, particularly in the perilous matter of interpreting religious meanings and ascribing religious beliefs to real people, as Watkins argues, we may not safely be able to escape the two-tier model, in a sense that the literate always need to find ways of closing down or glossing actions and reflections that might otherwise be open-ended and multivalent, as are relic-oriented religious practices par excellence. But we must at least try in our excavation or decompression of these stories, to get beyond belief and to find ways of interpreting diffuse forms of object-oriented authorisation of the miraculous.

Relic'ing in Twelfth-Century Miracle Narratives

In the remainder of this chapter I shall sketch out with the help of a few examples an approach to 'relic'ing' that considers three aspects of object-oriented activity: the magnetic force of relics; relic-oriented remembering and relic-mediated networking through gift-exchange. In practice these coalesced, but we shall consider them separately here.

Patrick Geary has noted that 'unlike other objects, the bare relic – a bone or a bit of dust – carries no fixed code or sign of its meaning as it moves from one community to another or from one period to a subsequent one'.[42] As he implies, there were few moments when relics were totally 'bare' in this way: they gathered personal biographies through their circulation; they were encased in composite and often decorative and valuable materials that had their own provenances; they were collected with the remains of other saints in relic collections and treasuries.[43] But when they were

---

[42] Patrick J. Geary, *Furta Sacra: Thefts of Relics in the Central Middle Ages* (Princeton, 1990), 5.

[43] Thomas Head, 'Art and artifice in Ottonian Trier', *Gesta*, 36 (1997), 65-82, and Cynthia Hahn, 'The meaning of early medieval treasuries', in *Reliquiare*

exposed to the religious, they often had the effect of flames to a moth. We have already seen examples of reckless monks and nuns punished for handling relics, and for attempting to keep fragments of relics. Thierry of Echternach, a contemporary of Guibert, explained the containment of relics in gold, silver and bejeweled reliquaries, as intended to represent the majesty of their content. They were also crucial in protecting the devotee from something they might otherwise, in the naked presence of the relic itself, find too powerful or disturbing to comprehend.[44] The effect he describes has a family resemblance to that version of fetishism defined by the anthropologist David Graeber as, the 'mistaking [of] the power of a history internalized in one's own desires, for a power intrinsic to the object itself'.[45]

The terrible power of relics to attract and, as we have seen, to destroy their religious handlers, is balanced by other stories of religious craving for relics satisfied through metaphors of eating and drinking in the energy emanating from relics. Arcoid, the author of the *Miracles of St Erkenwald*, for example, refers to miracles as heavenly sacraments (*caelestia sacramenta*), giving spiritual nourishment (*anime pabulum*), marvels (*magnalia*) that he exhorts the canons of his church 'lest pearls should seem to have been cast before swine' to 'take ... [as] a spiritual pattern of our salvation'.[46] When the monks of Sherborne learned about their saintly predecessor, Wulfsige, through their older brethren, 'the current brothers eagerly drank in these stories from their predecessors who knew the great father'.[47] Guibert's treatise contains the story of an

---

im Mittelalter, edited by Bruno Reudenbach and Gia Toussaint (Berlin, 2011), 1-20.

[44] Thiofrid of Echternach, *Flores Epytaphii Sanctorum*, edited by Michele C. Ferrari, Corpus Christianorum, Continuatio Medievalis, 133 (Turnhout, 1996), 39.

[45] David Graeber, *Toward an Anthropological Theory*, 115.

[46] *The Saint of London: The Life and Miracles of St. Erkenwald: Text and Translation*, edited and translated by E. Gordon Whatley (Binghampton, New York, 1989), 102-103, citing Romans 15:4.

[47] Rosalind Love, 'Life of Wulfsige of Sherborne by Goscelin of St Bertin: a new translation with introduction, appendix and notes', in *St Wulfsige and Sherborne: Essays to Celebrate the Millennium of the Benedictine Abbey 998-1998*, edited by Katherine Barker, David A. Hinton and Alan Hunt (Oxford, 2005), 102.

acolyte of the priests of Saint-Quentin, whose irreverent words addressed comically to a plaster image of the crucified Lord in the chancel of his church, 'Lord, do you want some of my bread', rebounded on him. The plaster image responded with the words, 'I shall shortly give you some of my bread', and Guibert reports that 'now the boy is buried before the image that made this promise to him'.[48] A telling food analogy crops up in Lection VI of *Cum orbita solis*, a brief treatise on miracles written by Sicard, Bishop of Cremona, in support of St Homobono's candidature for papal canonization in the late 1190s: 'as faith grows cool, wickedness abounds and the charity of many is cold. Then the supreme goodness of God repeats miracles, so that faith may be born and grow strong with the food of miracles'. This prepared the way, in the same paragraph, for a comparison of miracles with the supreme miracle of the Eucharist, 'what is more marvelous than that bread is changed into flesh and wine into blood?'.[49]

Relics and Mnemonic Practice

We can read and be grateful to the religious in Anglo-Norman England who increasingly felt writing down miracle stories was a superior means of storing memories for future retrieval. In his preface to the miracles of St Aethelthryth, Goscelin writes, 'we ought most carefully to search out their miracles and outward signs ... and lest they slip from memory, to record them most wisely in

---

[48] Vultis, ait, Domine, de pane meo? Cui ille evidentissime respondere dignatur 'Ego, ait, in proxime tibi de meo meo pane dabo', Qui his auditis morbo corripitur, et infra dies paucissimos suo quem brevi tenuerat exutus hominiculo, compos trabeae coelestia efficitur, et ante imaginem, quae id sibi spoponderat sepelitur. Guibert of Nogent, '*De sanctis et eorum pigneribus*', 92; Guibert of Nogent, '*Monodies' and 'On the Relics of Saints*', translated by McAlhany and Rubenstein, 200.

[49] For this translation see Brenda Bolton, 'Supporting the faith in medieval Rome', in *Signs, Wonders, Miracles: Representations of Divine Power in the Life of the Church*, edited by Kate Cooper and Jeremy Gregory, Studies in Church History, 41 (Woodbridge, 2005), 163. For twelfth-century developments in eucharistic theology and ritual see Miri Rubin, *Corpus Christi: The Eucharist in Late Medieval Culture* (Cambridge, 1991), 12-35 and Walker Bynum, *Christian Materiality*, 124-37.

books'.⁵⁰ But memories of the saints were transmitted in other ways. The religious did not give up oral forms of commemoration in doing so, the nuns at Wilton providing the following example of continued oral transmission: 'the chief lady of the monastery, Godiva ... and the other spiritual mothers ... as well as the things which they saw with their own eyes, declared confidently, with other appropriate evidence, those things which they heard from the venerable senior nuns, who ... saw the holy virgin herself'.⁵¹ These kinds of oral memories, held within religious communities are revealed in the narratives that fixed them for posterity.

But memories could also be more diffusely kept and transmitted through the use of objects originating in the everyday material lives of the laity. An interesting approach to this practice of remembering with objects is that of the anthropologist Karin Barber, who has worked on 'intentional forms' and processes of 'entextualization' in West African and other oral cultures. Her terms are remarkably close in usage to what the medieval historian Mary Carruthers calls memorial 'textualizing' in medieval literate culture, except that Barber applies them in much wider fields of oral, performative and object-oriented composition. A text can be any 'intentional form' lifted out of everyday interaction 'set up to be interpreted: as a challenge, a puzzle or a demand'.⁵²

One particular example of object-oriented intentionality was facilitated by the 'proverb custodian' of Akan-speaking Ghana who, like a patent officer, 'registered' newly coined sayings by means of objects brought to him and hung inside his house. Barber notes that these objects stood as provocation to the onlooker, posing 'a puzzle and a challenge',⁵³ acting as mnemonic invitations or

---

[50] Debemus perquirere ac recepta ne labantur a memoria sagacissime libris inserere. *Goscelin of Saint-Bertin: The Hagiography of the Female Saints of Ely*, 98-99.

[51] *Writing the Wilton Women*, 24. For the modern Latin edition see André Wilmart, 'La légendé de Ste Édith en prose et vers par la moine Goscelin', *Analecta Bollandiana*, 56 (1938), 36-37.

[52] Karin Barber, *The Anthropology of Texts, Persons and Publics Oral and Written in Africa and Beyond* (Cambridge, 2007), 5. Note the pioneering and related work on memory, gender, and material culture in medieval history of Elisabeth van Houts, *Memory and Gender in Medieval Europe, 900-1200* (London, 1999).

[53] Barber, *Anthropology of Texts*, 76.

prompts. What are they for? How did they get here? What do they mean? If asked, the custodian would offer his own memories of how the object came into his possession, recalling the personal story of the visitor who came to register the proverb, perhaps discussing the provenance or the meaning of the object, or the proverb it objectified, or even referring the questioner to the person who coined the new saying.

Through these 'intentional commemorative techniques' and exchanges, according to Barber, the objects are 'bathed in a sea of historical and contextual detail, which is not encoded within the object or the proverb, but is transmitted in another genre – the personal narrative – that runs alongside them'.[54] We might apply this approach to medieval miracle stories, in terms of the weaving of personal memories not into texts but into relics, that give us a glimpse of a micro-political economy of 'relic'ing' in which memories are 'narrated or performed into' bodily or secondary relics and other bespoke devotional objects.

For example, an Italian noblewoman, Benedicta of Tuscany, paid an extended visit to the shrine of St Erkenwald of London, during which time she prayed devoutly to the saint to restore function and form to her shriveled and paralyzed hand. When her prayers were answered, the woman herself, 'to encourage people to remember and reflect on so great a miracle, with sincere devotion, placed a hand made of wax on the tomb of the saint'.[55] A woman from Waer in Herfortshire, travelled to Canterbury and was partially cured by St Thomas of a condition that left her bent double. She was completely healed at Finchale by St Godric, on her return from a pilgrimage to St Andrew's in Scotland. The woman left her crutch and a candle above the altar (*cunctis videntibus ac mirantibus*).[56] Another woman from Witeburne left her crutch over the altar after a similar cure.[57] A certain prisoner (*captivus*) was

---

[54] Barber, *Anthropology of Texts*, 75-76.

[55] Ad memorian tanti miraculi recolendam, manum ceream super sancti tumulum sincera devotione apposuit. Gordon Whatley, *The Saint of London*, 129-33.

[56] Reginald of Durham, *Libellus de vita et miraculis S Godrici*, edited by Joseph Stevenson, Surtees Society, 20 (London, 1845), 376.

[57] Ibid., 371.

released from his chains when he visited the shrine of St Erkenwald. He was presented as a spectacle, and a peg for homily, with which people might reflect upon the chains of sin binding them from which they might hope for release in a life of devotion to God.[58] Philip de Bella Arbore, a penitent fratricidal knight of Lorraine, was relieved of his fetters at the shrine of St William of Norwich, 'releasing him from sin'.[59] A penitent who turned up at the shrine of St Modwenna was freed of iron bands around his belly and shoulder, which were suspended over the altar *pro memoria et testimonio*.[60] A servant of the saint caught in the act of theft on his feast day, escaped and fled to the altar of Ecgwin where his manacles fell from his hands, and he remained there giving thanks to the saint.[61]

Relics and Giving

The third form of relic-oriented activity I want to consider is gift-exchange. An interesting passage in Guibert's treatise begins with the following citation from Seneca's *De Beneficiis*: 'he who in return for another's generosity makes a payment according to value alone follows the example of merchants, while he who gives freely imitates God ... it is much more natural for God to offer a gift freely than to bestow a gift on someone based on whether he has earned it'.[62] Guibert frames this insight in terms of the faith people offer God. Seneca's notion of reciprocity and the commercial connotations of its defective forms are rendered in Christian terms by Guibert as a form of self-help, activated by God's will through Christ's recognition of someone's faith. Faith has power to move

---

[58] Gordon Whatley, *The Saint of London*, 117-19.
[59] Thomas of Monmouth, *The Life and Miracles of St William of Norwich*, edited and translated by Augustus Jessopp and Montague R. James (Cambridge, 1896), 13.
[60] Geoffrey of Burton, *The Life and Miracles of St Modwenna*, edited and translated by Robert Bartlett (Oxford, 2002), 191.
[61] *Chronicon abbatiae de Evesham ad annum 1418*, edited by William D. Macray (London, 1863), 63.
[62] Quia qui vicem alienae largitati restituit, mercatoribus exaequatur, qui autem gratuito impendit, Deum imitator. Guibert of Nogent, '*De sanctis et eorum pigneribus*', 92; Guibert of Nogent, '*Monodies' and 'On the Relics of Saints*', translated by McAlhany and Rubenstein, 200.

'he whose food is to do the will of his father', to permit those seeking cures to heal themselves through sharing in his salvation.

Twelfth-century miracle stories often emphasize the devotion, longing, contrition and emotional commitment manifest in those pilgrims cured at the shrines of their saints. But it is clear that pilgrims made sure they did not come empty handed to the shrines of saints. David Graeber's recent discussion of Mauss's classic work *The Gift* provides some insight into the micro-political dynamics of reciprocity that Mauss sought to articulate (but which are sometimes reduced into a trite formula as 'there is no such thing as a free gift'). A brief summary of these might help us to understand what we might be missing behind the numerous examples of gift-exchange provided by twelfth-century miracle narratives that we normatively describe as votive offerings. Graeber proposes four types of reciprocity emerging from Mauss's analysis: first, the open-exchange, in which everyone is chipping in and no-one is keeping score, an example being the family; the second, closed, balanced exchange, in which A gives B something and B immediately counter-gifts, mutual obligations thus cancelled out and equal status asserted (Seneca's market transaction or barter); the third, aggressive exchange or potlatch, in which a hierarchical relationship is asserted through agonistic destruction of goods, and finally, an open exchange with mild aggression in which a party within an open system feels they want to check the scoreboard by demanding acknowledgement for giving a gift, an example of which being the child rebelling against the parent.[63]

Our miracle stories' incorporation of gift exchange is represented as markers of intention in the form of a votive offering. William, a young man from France, was struck down in his London lodgings on the day of a procession of St Erkenwald. After three days he had wax eye castings placed on the rail suspended above St Erkenwald's shrine and 'the most precious illuminator, understood from within his tomb'.[64] Adam, the clerk of Yarmouth took with him to Norwich cathedral a candle measured to his height and breadth.[65] Alice, the daughter of a clerk of Essex was

---

[63] Graeber, *Toward an Anthropological Theory*, 217-28.
[64] Gordon Whatley, *The Saint of London*, 141.
[65] Thomas of Monmouth, *Life and Miracles*, 210.

advised in a dream by St James to buy a candle and take it to his shrine at Reading.⁶⁶ Gilbert, an ill pilgrim from the north who left Reading without a cure, was told in a dream to return and have a candle measured for him and await a cure.⁶⁷ William of Norwich made it explicit in a vision to one of his pilgrims that he liked candles.⁶⁸ Wulmar, returning to England from a pilgrimage to Rome, deposited marble and four rock crystals in the altar of St Edmund of Bury, that he had carried from Rome explained as 'offerings ... for the return of his health' (*oblato ... pro sua reversione salubri*).⁶⁹ A woman from Dover sent an offering, (*oblationem suam*) through the hands of messengers to the shrine of St Ecgwin, promising to give even more if she might be cured.⁷⁰ The practice of bending a penny to mark a pledge or thank offering (*devovere*), is documented for the miracles of St Cuthbert and St Godric.⁷¹

It is perhaps the fourth, attention-seeking, version of reciprocity that these examples most resemble. The objects chosen as votives were a mix of things that were often close to hand, commodities (candles, money, cloth) or valuable materials that might have particular symbolic and decorative value to the shrine (marble, rock crystal). These were removed from economic circulation by acts of personalisation on the part of the giver or their relatives. These acts we might imagine involved a degree of thought, craftsmanship and effort, as in the case of the man who made a presentation box for his wife to place the worm in that she vomited up when cured of

---

⁶⁶ 'Miracles of the hand of St James', edited and translated by Brian R. Kemp, *Berkshire Archaeological Journal*, 65 (1970), 9.

⁶⁷ 'Miracles of the hand of St James', 13.

⁶⁸ Thomas of Monmouth, *Life and Miracles*, 136-45.

⁶⁹ *Memorials of St Edmund's Abbey*, volume 1, 80-83. He had fallen into a trance for four days. Note the usefulness of marble and rock crystal in the making of reliquaries, Martina Bagnoli, 'The stuff of heaven: materials and craftsmanship in medieval reliquaries', in *Treasures of Heaven: Saints, Relics and Devotion in Medieval Europe*, edited by Martina Bagnoli et al. (London, 2011), 137-47.

⁷⁰ *Chronicon abbatiae de Evesham*, 62-63.

⁷¹ *Reginaldi monachi Dunelmensis, libellus de admirandis beati Cuthberti virtutibus*, edited by James Raine, Surtees Society, 1 (Durham, 1835), 231; Reginald of Durham, *Libellus de vita*, 410, 443; Vauchez, *Sainthood*, 453-59.

her illness by St Mildburg of Much Wenlock.⁷² They might even involve a significant artistic commission as in the case of Mabel le Bec who paid for the production of a reliquary into which the monks of Norwich Cathedral could place the slipper of St William.⁷³ They could involve having oneself measured to the length of a candlewick, or having the wax replica of a body part made. Or they could be the simple act of taking a penny from one's pocket and bending it, or being given a coin by a relative, as in the case of Ysembela, thrown out by her stepmother, but sent to a shrine by her aunt.⁷⁴

Conclusion

Commemoration, devotion and the desire to communicate with a saint through the exchange of a personalised token speak to a materiality of relic piety that encompasses and goes beyond hagiographical conventions and theological rationalisations of our sources, in ways that we would do well to explore if we want to appreciate the social significance of saints' cults. The point is that these acts of giving, of remembering and of projecting ones desires onto relics emerged from and modified the social lives of those who participated in them, beyond the focus of the miracles themselves, and in ways illustrative of object-oriented religion, not the textually interpreted version of it we see in miracle narratives. If nothing else, medieval relics offered opportunities for the evaluation and interpretation of actions and of objects and of object-oriented actions. While we may not see these practices in their entirety, they are sufficiently implicated in the sources for us to note their importance and take our cue from them in our attempts to glimpse the more diffuse social techniques and forms of expertise encompassing but extending among those who fostered saints' cults in everyday lived religion beyond the literate elite.

---

[72] Paul Antony Hayward, 'The *Miracula inventionis beate mylburge virginis* attributed to "the Lord Ato, Cardinal Bishop of Ostia"', *English Historical Review*, 114 (1999), 567-68.
[73] Yarrow, *Saints and their Communities*, 161.
[74] Yarrow, *Saints and their Communities*, 206-07.

MARIAN MIRACLES AND MARIAN LITURGIES IN THE BENEDICTINE TRADITION OF POST-CONQUEST ENGLAND

Kati Ihnat

In the century following the Norman Conquest, miracle literature in England emerged as one of the defining genres of monastic literary culture. The unique circumstances brought about by the military invasion and occupation of England by the Normans fostered a vivid interest in history writing in order to preserve the rich pre-Conquest religious culture, both to save it from being forgotten and to brief those ecclesiastical leaders newly arrived.[1] The lives and miracles of English saints were central to the historical memory of the particular institutions with which they were associated. Miracles attributed to relics acted as reminders of the religious heritage of individual churches and bestowed authority and legitimacy to claims of saintly patronage, crucial to a church's prestige. Recognizing the importance of the genre, Paul Hayward, Simon Yarrow and Rachel Koopmans, among others, have underscored the diverse rationales underlying the sudden enthusiasm for miracle-collecting at a time of significant social and cultural upheaval, variously emphasising miracles as loci for the negotiation of political and institutional identities, sources for understanding the construction of saints' cults, and textual remnants that conserved a predominantly oral tradition.[2] Within

---

[1] See, for example, Antonia Gransden, 'Traditionalism and continuity during the last century of Anglo-Saxon monasticism', *Journal of Ecclesiastical History*, 40 (1989), 159-207. For the rise of written culture in Anglo-Norman England more generally, see the standard work by Michael Clanchy, *From Memory to Written Record: England 1066-1307*, 3rd edn (Chichester, 2013).

[2] See most recently, Paul Antony Hayward, 'The cult of St Alban, Anglorum protomartyr, in Anglo-Saxon and Anglo-Norman England', in *More than a Memory: The Discourse of Martyrdom and the Construction of Christian Identity in the History of Christianity*, edited by Johan Leemans (Leuven, 2005), 169-

the 'change *vs.* continuity' debate that still occupies scholars of the Norman Conquest and its aftermath, the tremendous upsurge in written accounts of miracles is now acknowledged as an important testimony of the cultural shifts that marked the transition of the kingdom from Anglo-Saxon to Anglo-Norman rule.

All this scholarly activity has spared little attention for the miracles associated with the cult of one of Anglo-Saxon England's most prominent saints: the Virgin Mary.[3] Perhaps Mary's universality – she was not strictly speaking an English saint – and lack of any relic cult until the mid-twelfth century have made the cult seem less interesting to scholars of the period, despite the fact that the first collections of her miracles appeared in England in the early twelfth century. Perhaps the universal quality of these stories, drawn from many diverse sources and not limited to any one institution, has led scholars to believe they hold little value for local history. Whatever the reason, collections of Marian miracles have been relatively sidelined despite the considerable interest in miracle-collecting on the one hand and in the Marian cult on the other that we see in post-Conquest monastic culture. Marian miracles were instrumental for creating a hagiography of Mary similar to that of the Anglo-Saxon saints, particularly at institutions that boasted her patronage. Yet because Mary was fundamentally different from these saints, the subject matter of her miracles necessarily reflects different interests. The centrality of liturgical practices in the miracle accounts suggests that the emergence of such literature was tied up with the development of a Marian cult in which the liturgy had a primary role. This paper will therefore trace the presence of the liturgy in the miracles, exploring how these accounts reveal interest in forms of veneration, some of them novel, that were becoming increasingly expressive of Marian devotion, and suggest

99; Simon Yarrow, *Saints and their Communities: Miracle Stories in Twelfth-Century England* (Oxford, 2006); Rachel Koopmans, *Wonderful to Relate: Miracle Stories and Miracle Collecting in High Medieval England* (Philadelphia, 2011), and also Monika Otter, '1066: the moment of transition in two narratives of the Norman Conquest', *Speculum*, 74 (1999), 565-86.

[3] The importance of the Virgin Mary's cult was highlighted in a comprehensive, interdisciplinary study: Mary Clayton, *The Cult of the Virgin Mary in Anglo-Saxon England* (Cambridge, 1990).

that miracles were important tools for promoting such liturgical innovation.

Origins of the Marian Miracle Collections

Based on the extensive efforts of nineteenth-century philologists and codicologists to identify and catalogue manuscripts of Marian miracle collections, Richard Southern was the first to argue that the genre originated in twelfth-century England.[4] Led by the contents of the stories, combined with the English provenance of some of the earliest existing manuscripts, Southern was able to pinpoint the authors of the first three collections: Anselm, Abbot of Bury St Edmunds (d. 1148), Dominic, Prior of Evesham (d. *c.* 1130), and William, precentor of Malmesbury (d. 1143).[5] Although his arguments are compelling, Southern's desire to fix the collections to known individuals may have led him to over-emphasise their role as sole authors. The variety in style, subject matter and length of the many stories that made their way into the collections suggests the activity of numerous anonymous scribes actively shaping the volumes they were copying by adding, subtracting and altering miracles. For example, Southern took Chicago UL MS 147 to be a copy of Anselm's collection, although the stories in the second half are extremely diverse in style and form. They were likely added on to the first eighteen stories that constitute the core volume in stages. Southern nevertheless established the Marian miracles as

---

[4] Richard W. Southern, 'The English origins of the "Miracles of the Virgin"', *Medieval and Renaissance Studies*, 4 (1958), 176-216. Southern drew from the work of Adolfo Mussafia, *Studien zu den mittelalterlichen Marienlegenden*, 4 vols (Vienna, 1887-91); Carl Neuhaus, *Die Quellen zu Adgars Marienlegenden* (Aschersleben, 1882); Carl Neuhaus, *Die lateinischen Vorlagen zu den alt-französischen Adgar'schen Marien-Legenden* (Aschersleben, 1887); Henry L. D. Ward, *Catalogue of Romances in the Department of Manuscripts of the British Museum* (London, 1883) and the introduction of John of Garland, *Stella maris*, edited by Evelyn Faye Wilson (Cambridge, Massachusetts, 1946).

[5] William and Dominic's texts have been edited by José Maria Canal, while an extended version of Anselm's collection, found in Chicago: University Library 147, was transcribed by Elise Dexter. William of Malmesbury, *El libro 'De laudibus et miraculis Sanctae Mariae'*, edited by José Maria Canal (Rome, 1968); Dominic of Evesham, *'De miraculis Sanctae Mariae'*, edited by José Maria Canal, *Studium Legionense*, 39 (1998); *Miracula Sanctae Virginis Mariae*, edited by Elise F. Dexter (Madison, Wisconsin, 1927).

part of the rich monastic literary culture in England, and one he considered among the kingdom's greatest contributions to the 'twelfth-century Renaissance'.[6]

For the most part, studies of the Marian miracles have approached the collections from a text-critical approach, looking to identify further compilers, as well as the links between individual collections in order to establish *stemmae* of manuscripts.[7] A recent assessment of miracle literature by Rachel Koopmans has contextualized the first Marian miracle collections as part of a national literary trend. Discussing the Marian miracles only very briefly, Koopmans considers them together with the hagiographies and miracle collections of the Anglo-Saxon saints that became fashionable in post-Conquest England.[8] The prologues of the earliest Marian collections certainly support this approach. Anselm, Dominic and William all state that their efforts in collecting accounts of Mary's miracles were to fill a gap; other saints were the objects of hagiographical attention, so why not Mary, the patron saint of Bury, Evesham and Malmesbury? Anselm's prologue, which opens most subsequent collections, relates that, 'since the miracles of the saints are often recited in praise of God's omnipotence, who through them acts with divine clemency, how much more so should the actions of the blessed mother of God, Mary, be called to mind, which are all sweeter than honey?'[9] While Koopmans' rationale therefore applies equally to the Marian

---

[6] Richard, W. Southern, *The Making of the Middle Ages* (London, 1970), 236. Richard W. Southern, 'The place of England in the twelfth-century Renaissance', in *Medieval Humanism and Other Studies*, edited by Richard W. Southern (Oxford, 1970), 158-80. For a sceptical assessment of the genre's importance, see Rodney M. Thomson, 'England and the twelfth-century Renaissance', *Past and Present*, 101 (1983), 11.

[7] A very recent attempt to contribute to this process is the database of the Oxford Cantigas de Santa Maria project, which lists manuscripts and their contents for easy comparison: http://csm.mml.ox.ac.uk/?p=database [accessed 5 December 2011].

[8] Koopmans, *Wonderful to Relate*, 93 and 101.

[9] Ad omnipotentis dei laudem cum sepe recitentur sanctorum miracula que per eos egit divina clementia, maxime sancte dei genitricis Marie debent referri preconia, que sunt omni melle dulciora: *Miracula Sanctae Mariae*, 15. Both William and Dominic express very nearly the same in their prologues. Dominic of Evesham, *De miraculis*, 57 and William of Malmesbury, *De laudibus et miraculis*, 63.

miracles, she nevertheless tends to look at the genre from a literary standpoint. Miracles thus become textual traces recorded to preserve a lively oral tradition of miracle-storytelling, only to be filed away for posterity. This approach neglects the active role written miracle accounts had in performing devotion to the saint. Filling legendaries that would have been read from during the monastic office of Matins and at meal times, miracles were central to the liturgical celebration of the saint's feast day.

The importance of miracles for the liturgy did not stop there, and here the distinction between miracles performed by Mary and those by other saints becomes fundamental. Miracle stories described and prescribed the actions necessary for becoming the beneficiary of a saint's intervention, and in most cases, this included going on pilgrimage, worshipping at a shrine and making a donation to a religious institution. Mary was thought not to have left bodily remains on earth, apart from secondary relics, such as hair, milk and items of clothing.[10] In England, even these were not the focus of cult activity, and until the mid-twelfth century, there were no shrines of the kind found in France at Chartres, Laon and Rocamadour.[11] The Marian cult, as it was developed in post-Conquest England, emphasised other forms of devotional behaviour, and these became the main subject of the first collections of her miracles.

A survey of the stories in the earliest Marian collections highlights the prevalence of the liturgy as the primary means to secure Mary's mercy and miraculous aid. In Anselm's collection, eleven out of seventeen miracles involve identifiable practices: a prayer, a greeting, an antiphon, a Mass or a more elaborate office. Six of Dominic's fourteen miracles have the protagonist rewarded

---

[10] This had to do with the doctrine of Mary's bodily Assumption, which was the subject of considerable debate throughout the middle ages, but found important proponents in twelfth-century England such as Honorius Augustodunensis and William of Malmesbury. See Henry Mayr-Harting, 'The idea of the Assumption in the West, 800-1200', in *The Church and Mary*, edited by Robert N. Swanson, Studies in Church History, 39 (Woodbridge, 2004), 86-111.

[11] The earliest and most important Marian shrine at Walsingham probably dates from the mid-twelfth century, as argued by Clayton, *The Cult of the Virgin Mary*, 139-41.

for the same types of acts. William's extensive collection of fifty-one miracles has twenty-four miracles that feature a particular practice; the others involve Marian images and churches, and characters described as having a general devotion to Mary. Of the eighteen most popular miracles added to subsequent collections, seven involve commemoration via feast days, prayers, offices and Masses.[12] Many of these accounts were preserved in twelfth-century copies of the collections, further stressing their relevance over and above those involving pilgrimage to a church, worship of a relic or icon, or just general devotion to the Virgin, which appear with far less frequency.[13] We must be wary of such statistical analysis, however. Making sense of miracle collections by tallying up the various themes and features can be misleading, as it does not necessarily reflect the popularity of individual stories that went on to circulate in sermons and through oral transmission. The frequency with which liturgical practices feature nevertheless allows a preliminary grasp of the relative importance of the liturgy for the twelfth-century compilers of Marian miracles, something that distinguishes them from miracles associated with locally-based saints.

The importance of liturgical practice in the Marian miracle collections was recognised by Benedicta Ward in her wide-ranging study of the miraculous in medieval religious culture.[14] Unlike studies before and since, hers gives importance to the devotions described in the miracles, enumerating them not only in the collections with origins in England, but also the local collections

---

[12] These are found, for example, in a complete series in a mid-twelfth-century manuscript, Chicago: University Library MS 147, but not in consistent order or number in most other manuscripts.

[13] The manuscripts consulted containing these stories include, London: British Library, Additional MS 35112; Arundel MS 346; Cotton Cleopatra MS C. x; Egerton MS 2947. London: Lambeth Palace Library, MS 214. Paris: Bibliothèque Nationale, lat. MS 2672; lat. MS 2769; lat. MS 2873; lat. MS 3809A; lat. MS 12169; lat. MS 12606; lat. MS 14463; lat. MS 18168. Cambridge: Corpus Christi College, MS 42. Oxford: Bodleian Library, Canon. Liturg. MS 325 and Laud Misc. MS 410. Chicago: University Library, MS 147 (formerly Phillips 25142). Copenhagen: Thott MS 26, 8; Thott MS 128, 2.

[14] Benedicta Ward, *Miracles and the Medieval Mind: Theory, Record and Event* (London, 1982).

from French churches and abbeys, such as Coutances, Laon, Chartres, Rocamadour and Soissons.[15] She distinguishes between the two types by contrasting the pilgrimages and donations to particular shrines that dominate the French type with the more general liturgical practices described in the English collections that could be celebrated in any church. Ward's study thus treats these latter practices as timeless, discussing them as 'universal devotions, untethered by place'.[16] Without reference to the historical context in which the texts were written, however, it remains to be seen what motivated their redaction precisely at this time by English monks. If the local French collections were recorded to foster pilgrimage, as we have come to expect from records of miracles of the saints, what would explain the drive of English monks to depict liturgical practices that were so widespread?

In order to answer this question, it becomes essential to discuss both the collections and the individual stories they contain as a feature of a particular devotional milieu. By examining some of the most common practices described in the miracle collections and comparing them to liturgical practice in the same monastic context in which the miracles were recorded, we can begin to understand how liturgy and miracle functioned together. Taking each practice separately and tracing its devotional history in England reveals a close relation between the establishment of increasingly elaborate forms of Marian worship in the early-twelfth century and their treatment in miracle accounts from the same period.[17] Instead of

---

[15] These collections promote shrines at particular institutions, on which see Gabriela Signori, 'La bienheureuse polysémie, miracles et pèlerinages à la Vierge: pouvoir thaumaturgique et modèles pastoraux (X^e-XIIe siècles)', in *Marie: Le Culte de la Vierge dans la société médiévale*, edited by Dominique Iogna-Prat, Éric Palazzo and Daniel Russo (Paris, 1996), 591-617, and *The Miracles of Our Lady of Rocamadour: Analysis and Translation*, edited and translated by Marcus Bull (Woodbridge, 1999).

[16] Ward, *Miracles and the Medieval Mind*, 162.

[17] The development of the Marian cult in Anglo-Norman England has increasingly been underscored, for example by Antonia Gransden, 'The cult of St Mary at Beodricisworth and then in Bury St Edmunds Abbey to *c.* 1150', *Journal of Ecclesiastical History*, 55 (2004), 627-53, and Nigel Morgan, 'Texts and images of Marian devotion in English twelfth-century monasticism, and their influence on the secular church', in *Monasteries and Society in Medieval Britain: Proceedings of the 1994 Harlaxton Symposium*, edited by Benjamin Thompson (Stamford, 1999), 117-36.

encouraging behaviour more typically associated with saints' cults, such as pilgrimage, here miracles come across as *apologiae* for novel liturgical practice, defending and supporting Mary's celebration in the liturgy in a period that saw her dramatic rise to prominence. The interaction between miracle and liturgy therefore ultimately helps unlock the genesis of the Marian miracle genre as an integral feature of Marian devotion in post-Conquest England.

Prayers, Antiphons and Masses

Prayer was clearly one of the foremost means to garner a miracle from the Virgin. While not reduced to the context of the liturgy, the 'Hail Mary' is worth considering here because of its frequent appearance in the miracles, some of which tie the prayer explicitly to the environment in which they were first written. The widespread appeal of the *Ave Maria* is reflected in its ability to save a number of people from all walks of life, including a fornicating sacristan, a sinful canon of Chartres cathedral, and a peasant who impinges on monastery land in order to expand his own.[18] A story about Eulalia, the abbess of Shaftesbury (d. 1106), nevertheless brings the Hail Mary into a distinctly English monastic context. The account describes how she is urged by Mary to say the greeting more slowly and solemnly, a practice the abbess later institutes in her convent.[19] After relating the miracle, the narrator of Eulalia's story then addresses his brothers directly, encouraging them to follow suit: 'and we, dearest brothers (who are not worthy to call ourselves her [Mary's] servants), if we aim to celebrate our service to her according to her will after this warning, I believe that we brothers must do what that holy woman was worthy of doing in

---

[18] These are all found in the vast majority of manuscripts listed above in note 13.

[19] 'I advise you that if you wish to devote yourself to doing me better service, and thereby please me, not to pronounce it so quickly ... and she [Eulalia] instituted the third part to be sung more solemnly and with great assiduity from this time forward'. Sed moneo te ut si illa que mihi impendis servitia tibi vis magis proficere, et mihi placere, tunc noli amodo ea tam velociter pronuntiare ... Tertiam cum magna diligentia amodo cantare morosius instituerat: *Miracula Sanctae Mariae*, 36. Giles Constable has indicated the emphasis placed on the proper, sincere recitation of Psalms by twelfth-century reformers. Giles Constable, *The Reformation of the Twelfth Century* (Cambridge, 1996), 206.

eternal beatitude'.[20] The story is told on the authority of a monk at Bec, suggesting that it was redacted by someone in the circle of Archbishop Anselm of Canterbury (d. 1109), who corresponded frequently with Eulalia and was also the uncle of Anselm of Bury, one of the earliest compilers.[21] Although the Hail Mary had a lengthy history, prescribed in the earliest Benedictine Rule and found in the liturgies of all Marian feast days and celebrations, the story of Eulalia would have brought the prayer into a recognisable context and made the message about sincere, thoughtful practice all the more poignant by the familiarity of the characters. The story's popularity in English manuscripts of miracle collections certainly suggests the practice held special significance for monastic communities in England.[22]

William of Malmesbury's story about the reward St Dunstan (d. 988) received for building a church in honour of Mary has a similar degree of local relevance. The Archbishop's efforts merited him the miracle of seeing Mary herself lead a choir of virgins singing the fifth-century hymn *Cantemus, Domino, sociae, cantemus honorem* in that same church.[23] Dunstan is urged to participate, and sings the antiphon *O rex gloriae, nate Maria virgine, salva genus christianorum in hac terra peregrinantium*.[24] The original *O rex gloriae* does not

---

[20] Et nos fratres karissimi, qui digni non summus ut illius vocemur servi, si eius servicium post hanc admonitionem, iuxta illius voluntate celebrare studuerimus, credo quod illius sanctimonialis feminae fratres nos in eterna beatitudine dignabitur facere: *Miracula Sanctae Mariae*, 36.

[21] Southern, 'The English origins', 190.

[22] See, for example: Cambridge: Corpus Christi College, MS 42; London: British Library, MS Cotton Cleopatra C. x. and MS Egerton 2947. Chicago: University Library, MS 147 and Paris, Bibliothéque Nationale, MS Lat. 2873. Though French in provenance, these texts contain a number of stories with English settings including Eulalia's account and were likely based on an English source.

[23] For the full text, see *Analecta Hymnica*, edited by Clemens Blume and Guido M. Dreves, volume 50 (Leipzig, 1886), 53.

[24] This account seems to be an amalgamation of two miracles in both William and Osbern's *Vitae* of Dunstan. *Memorials of Saint Dunstan, Archbishop of Canterbury*, edited by John Capgrave and William Stubbs, Rolls Series, 63 (London, 1874), 117-19. William of Malmesbury, *Saints' Lives*, 165-304. I was unable to find the hymn either in CANTUS database [http://cantusdatabase.org/] or in *Analecta hymnica medii aevi*, edited by G. M. Drèves, 55 vols (Leipzig, 1886-1922).

contain the reference to Mary, indicating that in redacting the miracle, William adapted the hymn Dunstan sang in an effort to make the antiphon relevant to the Marian cult, or alternatively, that by the time William recorded the story, the antiphon had come to incorporate the Virgin. The choir of virgins, with Mary as their leader, appear again in William's story about a church built at Bury St Edmunds at her request, although this time without the antiphon; perhaps this is because the protagonist is a rustic who cannot understand the 'mysterious mumbling' (*arcani murmuris*) coming from the church in which he finds her.[25] The stories share the idea that wherever Mary feels she is adequately honoured, particularly through the dedication of a church, she appears to perform the liturgy herself, here in specifically English settings.

Even without the construction of edifices in her honour, the singing of antiphons and responsories by Mary's followers had the power to secure her mercy. In a story by William of Malmesbury, a nun whose penance remains unfinished is nevertheless saved by the Virgin, thanks to frequent repetition of the Hail Mary and the antiphon *Gaude Dei genitrix*.[26] This same antiphon, sung daily, was also said to have saved a cleric from Chartres.[27] William comments that singing it is a way of remembering Mary's continual presence.[28] Both stories were likely inspired by the tale of the Five Gaudes, found in Anselm's original collection. In this case, the antiphon sung by the clerical protagonist is written out in its entirety.[29] Does this level of detail indicate that those hearing the miracle account would not have been familiar with the antiphon?

---

[25] William of Malmesbury, *De laudibus et miraculis*, 142.

[26] William of Malmesbury, *De laudibus et miraculis*, 156.

[27] William of Malmesbury, *De laudibus et miraculis*, 115-17.

[28] Imperaverat enim et persuaserat suae opinioni, ut dominam numquam putans absentem, semper imaginaretur praesentem, ut eius reverentiae intuitu, non solum se ad illecebras non exponeret, sed etiam ab illicitis temperaret. William of Malmesbury, *De laudibus et miraculis*, 116.

[29] Gaude dei genitrix, virgo immaculate/ Gaude que gaudium ab angelo suscepisti. /Gaude que genuisti eterni luminis claritatem/ Gaude mater/ Gaude sancta dei genitrix virgo/ Tu sola mater innupta, te laudat omnis factura genitricem virgo/ Tu sola mater innupta, te laudat omnis factura genitricem lucis, / Sis pro nobis quasi perpetua interventrix. *Miracula Sanctae Mariae*, 19.

The story is found in Peter Damian's (d. 1072) *De variis apparitionibus et miraculis*, which also contains the full text, but the antiphon originated a century earlier.[30] It may not have become widespread until much later, however, as it is first attested in England in a manuscript from Christ Church, Canterbury dated to the mid-eleventh century.[31] In this particular manuscript, it is incorporated into the hymn *Ave mater advocati*, which was later attributed to Anselm of Canterbury.[32] As a result, the antiphon's profile was no doubt raised such that its subject matter was subsequently expanded upon in the treatise, *De excellentia beata Mariae*, written by Anselm's biographer, Eadmer (d. c. 1130).[33]

Not to be confused with the *Gaude dei genitrix*, the responsory *Gaude Maria virgo* is the subject of a miracle involving a monk of Evesham that appears in both Dominic's and William's collections.[34] The soul of the monk is attacked by devils, but he is saved through singing the *Gaude Maria virgo*, whose text is as follows: 'Rejoice Mary, virgin, you alone opposed all heresies, you who believed the words of the Archangel Gabriel. Then the virgin gave birth to man and God and remained a virgin after the birth'.[35] The responsory dates back to the ninth century, but the earliest

---

[30] Petrus Damiani, '*De variis apparitionibus et miraculis*', *Patrologia Latina*, edited by Jacques P. Migne, volume 145 (1853), 588.

[31] London: British Library, MS Cotton Tiberius A. iii, fol. 111. While limited in its scope, the CANTUS database contains only 15 entries for the antiphon, mostly from the fourteenth century or later.

[32] Edward S. Dewick has dated it to sometime between 1032 and 1050. Edward S. Dewick, *Facsimiles of Horae de Beata Maria Virgine from English MSS of the Eleventh Century* (London, 1902), xiv.

[33] Eadmer of Canterbury, '*De excellentia beatae Mariae*', *Patrologia Latina*, edited by Jacques P. Migne, volume 159 (1853), 557-80. On which, see Richard W. Southern, *Saint Anselm and his Biographer: A Study of Monastic Life and Thought* (Cambridge, 1966), 289-90.

[34] William of Malmesbury, *De laudibus et miraculis*, 109.

[35] Gaude Maria virgo cunctas hereses sola interemisti que gabrielis archangeli dictis credidisti. Dum virgo domini et hominem genuisti et post partum virgo inviolata permansisti. For a history of the responsory and the antiphon drawn from it, see Louis Brou, 'Marie "Destructrice de toutes les hérésies" et la belle légende du répons *Gaude Maria Virgo*', *Ephemerides liturgicae* (1948), 321-53.

example in England is in the eleventh-century Winchester Troper.[36] It would eventually become, along with the *Gaude dei genitrix*, a fixture of Marian liturgies, one of the three closing texts of the Matins office. The inclusion of the full liturgical text in the story of the monk of Evesham suggests that it was featuring in English monastic liturgies by the early twelfth century.

A Mass said in honour of the Virgin is the subject of several miracle stories connected with English contexts that suggests it was of special interest for the early compilers. In a story rich in historical detail, said to have been told by Edricus, Prior of Chertsey, Leofric, a monk of Westminster Abbey desires to take over the abbacy of Chertsey against the wishes of his abbot.[37] The King's decision to give him the post regardless is met with great displeasure on the part of the monks of Westminster and Leofric is exiled to the abbey of Dol in Brittany. He is ultimately redeemed for his disobedience thanks to the one or two weekly Masses he performed in honour of Mary.[38] The practice originated with Alcuin of York (d. 804), who popularized a weekly Mass for Mary on Saturdays throughout Europe.[39] Perhaps this was the same Mass that features both in Anselm's and William's collections in a story about a priest who knew only one Mass and was therefore removed by his bishop, only to be reinstated at Mary's own insistence. This miracle would have stressed the benefits of daily recitation of a Marian Mass, which is described as *De Beata* with the introit *Salve*

---

[36] The Winchester manuscript is Cambridge: Corpus Christi College, MS 473, fol. 194. Michel Huglo, 'Remarks on the alleluia and responsory series in the Winchester Troper', in *Music in the Medieval English Liturgy: Plainsong and Medieval Music Society Centennial Essays*, edited by Susan Rankin and David Hiley (Oxford, 1993), 54.

[37] No abbot named Leofric appears in David Knowles, Christopher N. L. Brooke, Vera C. M. London, *The Heads of Religious Houses: England and Wales, 940-1216*, 2nd edn (Cambridge, 2001), 38.

[38] *Miracula Sanctae Mariae*, 52.

[39] Éric Palazzo, 'Le rôle de Libelli dans la pratique liturgique du haut moyen âge: histoire et typologie', *Revue Mabillon*, nouvelle série, 1 (1990), 25, and Dominique Iogna-Prat, 'Le Culte de la Vierge sous le règne de Charles le Chauve', in *Marie: le Culte de la Vierge dans la société médiévale*, edited by Dominique Iogna-Prat, Éric Palazzo and Daniel Russo (Paris, 1996), 80-81.

sancta parens.⁴⁰ A missal from St Augustine's, Canterbury, from the eleventh century, features this Mass at the end of the Sanctorale; its placement here suggests it was intended as a general Marian Mass not reserved for any specific feast day.⁴¹ The same Mass appears under the rubric *In veneratione Sancte Marie* in a twelfth-century sacramentary from St Albans, indicating that it too was performed whenever a Marian Mass was required.⁴²

The weekly Marian Mass on Saturday is also the subject of a popular miracle story added soon after the original collections had begun to circulate.⁴³ The tone and form of the text depart significantly from other stories in that it is more an apologia for the practice than an actual miracle account; it was in all likelihood originally a sermon with a short miracle account at its conclusion.⁴⁴ The text's main aim is to defend the expansion of the Marian Mass into a full commemorative office replacing the normal liturgical hours, claiming that 'it is proper for the sons of the church to celebrate by a solemn office, the solemn memory of the Holy Virgin Mary, since it is naturally conceded to many of the saints with a certain special dignity of familiarity', as if to say that Mary ought to be venerated with the same feeling as local saints.⁴⁵ The homiliarist urges that Mary be commemorated in this way not only on special feast days, but every Saturday, which should be universally dedicated to her:

> Many in the ecclesiastical sphere, though not all are able to, have chosen one day in the week to honour the Virgin mother. Would not

---

⁴⁰ William identifies the introit's composer as Sedulius (fl. *c.* 450) in his version. The full text of the *Salve sancta parens* is found in *Patrologia Latina*, edited by Jacques P. Migne, volume 19 (1846), 599-600. William of Malmesbury, *De laudibus et miraculis*, 124.

⁴¹ Cambridge: Corpus Christi College, MS 270, fols 139-139v.

⁴² Oxford: Bodleian Library, Rawl. Liturg. C, fol. 138v.

⁴³ An early exemplar is Chicago: University Library, MS 147, others include: Paris: Bibliothèque Nationale, MS Lat. 2672; Copenhagen, Thott 26, 8°; London: British Library, MS Cotton Cleopatra C. x.

⁴⁴ It appears explicitly as a sermon (*Sermo quare in Sabbatis fit memoria b. Marie*) in the twelfth-century miracle collection from Saint-Martin, Tournai, in London: British Library, MS Additional 35112.

⁴⁵ Sollempnem memoriam sancte Marie virginis, matris domini, decet filios ecclesie sollempni officio celebrare, quippe cum multis sanctorum concessum sit quadam spetiali dignitate familiaritatis. *Miracula Sanctae Mariae*, 48.

the feast day that best suits Mary be the seventh from the Sabbath [i.e. Saturday], which is a day free from the work of the other six days? ... Therefore on this day, many devotees, burning with zeal in gratitude of Mary, perform solemn service to the gracious mother. But lest a commemoration by single hours not tire them, it should be confirmed in the meantime by the authority of a synod that a Mass be sung, not without the *Gloria in excelsis deo*. And they prove this by reason, taking up an argument from a lesser situation: if a king or emperor should arrive, they ask, which church would not defer from its usual activities, adorning the front of the temple with golden crowns, and thuribles and other things for a procession? Therefore if the Paschal solemnities are renewed when earthly princes are present, it is most justified and pious that the Lady of the world, the glorious Mary, should be honoured on her Sabbath with a solemn office, in honour of the son who loves and honours his good mother. Therefore, in order that those who do not show themselves to do it properly might not be called foolish, let us perform *all the festivities* on Saturday, Mary's day.[46]

The homilist then concludes with a miracle of an image of Mary in Constantinople whose veil is miraculously raised every Saturday, much like the miracle of the Holy Sepulchre.

The text presents an interesting problem. It refers to a time when the degree to which Mary was thought to deserve celebration on Saturday was under debate. A synod or council is credited with the decision that a Mass was sufficient, although committed Marian devotees supported the adoption of a more extensive votive

---

[46] Plures in mundo ecclesie, quia non possunt omnes, elegerunt vel unam in ebdomada diem in tantae virginis matris honore. Que autem dies sic festiva Mariam deceret, quam septima sabbati, liberata ab omni senario opere diei? ... Igitur, in hac die multi fideles accensi zelo Marie ad gratiam reddunt sollempne servitium gratiose matri, sed ne fastidium generet festivitas per singulas horas, donec et illud confirmet sinodalis auctoritas missam tantum cantare sollempniter, nec sine gloria in excelsis deo. Et hoc probant ratione sumentes argumentum de minore. Si rex, inquiunt, vel imperator advenerit, que ecclesia est que non statim solitas procrastinet ferias, faciem templi coronis aureis adornans, thuribulis et ceteris ad processionem ordinatis? Igitur si ad terreni principis presentiam quodammodo renovatur pachalis sollempnitas, dignum et religiosum valde est ut mundi domina gloriosa Maria in suo sabbato honoretur sollempni officio, ad filii honorem qui diligit et honorat bonam matrem. Iam vero ne dicant insipientes apud se non recte confitantes, quiescere faciamus omnes festos dies Marie a sabbato. *Miracula Sanctae Mariae*, 50.

office. A context of monastic reform seems likely for such a discussion, although where and when this may have taken place is left unclear in the sermon. It is possible that such a question was tabled at the synodal council summoned *circa* 970 for the reform of England's monasteries under the aegis of King Edgar. Led by three prominent reformers (Dunstan, Archbishop of Canterbury, Oswald, Bishop of Worcester, and Aethelwold, Bishop of Winchester), the council resulted in the redaction of a monastic rule, the *Regularis Concordia*, in which the celebration of a Marian Mass on Saturdays is stipulated.[47] Among the leaders, Aethelwold was reputed to have been so personally devoted to the Virgin that he performed a daily votive office in her honour.[48] Perhaps someone in his circle composed the Saturday sermon to support the adoption of a full votive office in place of the Mass. If so, the arguments put forward were eventually successful, since by the end of the eleventh century a full office for Saturdays was copied in a liturgical manuscript that belonged to Wulfstan, Bishop of Worcester, *circa* 1065.[49] The practice's roots in the late tenth-century reform could additionally explain the sermon's incorporation into the twelfth-century miracle collections, as monks in the post-Conquest period looked back nostalgically at what they saw as the 'Golden Age' of English monasticism.[50] While it remains difficult to draw conclusions about whether the debate continued into the twelfth century, the scribe's decision to copy the sermon in its full form instead of simply extracting the miracle at the very end, gives some hint that the practice may have remained contentious.

---

[47] *Regularis Concordia: The Monastic Agreement*, edited and translated by Thomas Symons (London, 1953), x.

[48] Helene Scheck, *Reform and Resistance: Formations of Female Subjectivity in Early Medieval Ecclesiastical Culture* (Albany, 2008), 97. Many ecclesiastical establishments, in addition to being placed under a monastic rule, were rededicated to the Virgin in this period. For this, see Clayton, *The Cult of the Virgin Mary*, 128-29, and Alison Binns, *Dedications of Monastic Houses in England and Wales, 1066-1216* (Woodbridge, 1989), 18-27.

[49] For a transcription of this office, see Sally Elizabeth Roper, *Medieval English Benedictine Liturgy: Studies in the Formation, Structure and Content of the Monastic Votive Office, c. 950-1540* (New York, 1993), 243.

[50] On this, see Gransden, 'Traditionalism and continuity', 159-207.

The Little Office: Daily Votive Commemoration of Mary

From weekly to daily practice, the extent to which Mary was seen to deserve full liturgical observance is demonstrated by the large number of miracle accounts that depict the practice of honouring Mary with a daily liturgical *cursus* following each of the canonical hours, i.e. the Little Office or Hours of the Virgin.[51] In a story in Anselm's collection, Jerome of Pavia is described as an upstanding cleric who 'tried to please the mother of God, either by greeting her, by singing her hours, or by performing many different types of service in her honour'.[52] This is also the case in the tale of the prior of St. Saviour in Pavia, in which an otherwise wicked prior sings her praises at every liturgical hour.[53] In a story redacted by William of Malmesbury, a cleric of Chartres recites the Hours of Mary secretly, and she subsequently defends him in spite of his avaricious tendencies.[54] In another, a monk receives the gift of Mary's milk and has the Ave written on his tongue because he had the habit of reciting the Little Office privately, alternately kneeling, standing and lying down so as not to lose strength; this gives valuable indications as to the considerable length of time such a practice would have required, and the personal piety it was thought to express.[55]

The most famous of the Little Office stories is the *Cleric of Pisa*, found in both Anselm's and William's collections. A cleric devoted

---

[51] For a study of votive offices in English monastic culture, among them the Little Office, see Roper, *Medieval English Benedictine Liturgy*.

[52] Qui sancte dei genitrici placere studebat, vel salutando, vel horas eius canendo, vel etiam multis formis servicium eius agendo. *Miracula Sanctae Mariae*, 28.

[53] Sed quamvis ita videretur irreligiosus, sanctam Mariam matrem domini, non parum, diligens, singulis horis laudes dei eiusque canebat. Et dum eas caneret, semper stabat, nec ullatenus sedere volebat. *Miracula Sanctae Mariae*, 27.

[54] Nihilo tamen segnius vel remissiori officio sanctae Mariae horas cantabat, vel etiam intranseunter salutabat? William of Malmesbury, *De laudibus et miraculis*, 114-17.

[55] Ille eas undecumque compilatas, post horas canonicas in ecclesia, abscedentibus ceteris, decantabat. Id diebus, id noctibus indefesse concinnabat, saepe stans, saepius genibus flexis orans, numquam sedens, vel iacens, ne virtutem orationis eviraret mollities corporis. William of Malmesbury, *De laudibus et miraculis*, 83-84.

to the Virgin enough that he 'daily sings the hours in her honour, which was done very rarely in that time', is married off by his family, but after he sneaks away from the wedding to perform the liturgical devotion one last time, Mary appears to him in a jealous rage; terrified, he jumps out of his marriage bed presumably to return to Mary's service.[56] In a related story, *Love by Black Arts*, a cleric who made a pact with the devil in order to secure his beloved, continues to sing the Little Office, yet is cut short on his wedding day when Mary appears in a vision to remind him of his devotion to her; he promptly has the marriage dissolved.[57] Although there is no indication given as to the time in which the events are set, the fact that in all of the stories the Little Office is performed privately – at times in secret – is evidence that it may have been a practice associated with extreme personal devotion to the Virgin when the miracle narratives were first redacted.

This private nature of the Little Office is supported by stories in both Dominic and William's collections that describe the practice's origins. Dominic of Evesham includes a story about a pope who is chastised for his lax observance and consequently institutes the recitation of the Little Office by a single cleric in his service, in addition to the Saturday votive commemoration.[58] In a tale that is generally attributed to the abbot of Cluny, Odo, about a monk to whom Mary reveals herself as *mater misericordiae*, William describes the transition of the practice from private to communal celebration, placing it at Cluny:

---

[56] Hic sicuti de pluribus retulimus, sancte virgine Marie mundi regine, servitium devota mente reddebat, horasque diei que tunc temporis a paucissimis dicebantur, in eius honorem decantabat. *Miracula Sanctae Mariae*, 30. In William's version, he is said to have recited the Office privately: Pise eius privatas horas, ipse privata officia continuabat. William of Malmesbury, *De laudibus et miraculis*, 117.

[57] Mary recognises his efforts, saying: 'ego sum Maria, de qua cantabas horam'. William of Malmesbury, *De laudibus et miraculis*, 120-21.

[58] Constituit et unusquique clericus ordinatus sive monachus per singulos dies horas sanctae Mariae decantaret. Adiunxit etiam hanc institutionem ut in singulis hebdomadibus semper in sabbato commemoratio ipsius santissimae virginitatis ac fecunditatis fieret, quemadmodum in dominica fit commemoratio resurrectionis filii sui. Dominic of Evesham, *De miraculis*, 277.

> From that point on, in all of its communities which have completely filled the Latin world, they were not content to perform a private office, individually, but promoted a public office according to their customs, by praises sung after the hours. They convinced one of them to teach the office of Complines openly, which they thought should not be neglected by whosoever professed himself of the same service to Mary as them. I believe it is not to be slighted but extolled, because every occasion to apply oneself more devoutly to her service is to be embraced.[59]

The reference to Complines as a specifically Marian hour is also found in a story by Dominic and in numerous other anonymous collections, in which Mary appears to a monk to correct his liturgical performance.[60] But William's commentary on the practice's evolution from private to communal hints at opposition. Much like the defense of the extended Saturday office in the sermon discussed above, William attributes miraculous results to a practice he implies was not widely performed. Reference to Cluny sounds very much like an attempt on William's part to provide a precedent for the practice's adoption and lend it the prestige it seems to have lacked, which would explain the frequency with which the Hours of the Virgin appear in the miracles.

Was William correct in tracing the origins of the Little Office to Cluny, that font of monastic reform since the early tenth century? Some continental houses have evidence of a communal Little Office by the mid- to late-tenth century: St Gall, Satin-Maximin in Trier and Augsburg, for example.[61] As far as scholars have been able to ascertain, however, the practice of the Little Office was adopted

---

[59] Unde coenobii monachi, tanto usque ad hunc diem dominam communem venerantur honore, ut nihil supra. Denique in omnibus congregationibus suis, quae per orbem latinum amplissime porriguntur, non contenti singulorum clandestino officio, publico eam in conventionibus suis extollunt, horarum praeconio. Persuaserunt sibi ipsam conspicue suorum cuidam visam completorium docuisse, quod necnon negligendum arbitrantur, quicumque familiarem illi famulatum profitentur. Nec hoc insultans, immo exsultans dico, quia amplectenda est omnis occasio, qua illius quis devotius applicetur famulitio. William of Malmesbury, *De laudibus et miraculis*, 105.

[60] The entire office is described by Mary herself in this story, with every incipit of every liturgical text included. *Miracula Sanctae Mariae*, 15. Dominic of Evesham, *De miraculis*, 278.

[61] Kassius Hallinger, 'Neue Fragen der Reformgeschichtlichen Forschung', in *Archiv für mittelrheinische Kirchengeschichte*, 9 (1957), 1-32, at 23.

at Cluny only in the latter half of the eleventh century, possibly thanks to the abbot Hugh.[62] The customaries produced in the late eleventh century by the monks Bernard and Ulrich both contain references to a Little Office. Ulrich's customary, made *circa* 1060, has an intriguing instruction that during the baking of the host, the monk in charge should recite the Psalmody and additionally the Hours of the Virgin, if desired.[63]

Despite William's claims in his miracle account, there is liturgical evidence of a practice of the Little Office in England that predates any Cluniac equivalent. According to Orderic Vitalis (d. *c.* 1142), borrowing from Wulfstan of Winchester (fl. *c.* 1000), Aethelwold of Winchester is meant to have recited the Little Office after each of the canonical hours. Mary Clayton has identified an existing office for Vespers as part of this very practice, perhaps written by Aethelwold himself.[64] If not this precise text, the earliest complete offices are also found in English manuscripts.[65] A full office, from Matins to Compline, is appended to a collection of

---

[62] Ibid., and Barbara Rosenwein, 'Feudal war and monastic peace: Cluniac liturgy as ritual aggression', *Viator*, 2 (1971), 129-57, at 139.

[63] Canunt psalmodiam quae remansit, et, si voluerint, horas de S. Maria. Ulrich Cluniacensis, '*Antiquiores consuetudines cluniacensis monasterii*', *Patrologia Latina*, edited by Jacques P. Migne, volume 149 (1853), 758. For the liturgical contents of the customaries more generally – albeit without mention to the Little Office – see Susan Boynton, 'The Customaries of Bernard and Ulrich as liturgical sources', in *From Dead of Night to End of Day: The Medieval Customs of Cluny*, edited by Isabelle Cochelin and Susan Boynton (Turnhout, 2005), 109-30. For Marian devotion at Cluny, see Dominique Iogna-Prat, 'Politische Aspekte der Marienverehrung in Cluny um das Jahr 1000', in *Maria in der Welt: Marienverehrung im Kontext der Sozialgeschichte 10-18 Jahrhundert*, edited by Claudia Opitz, Hedwig Röckelein, Gabriela Signori and Guy P. Marchal (Zürich, 1993), 243-51 and Carolyn Marino Malone, 'Interprétation des pratiques liturgiques à Saint-Bénigne de Dijon d'après ses coutumiers d'inspiration clunisienne', in *From Dead of Night to End of Day: The Medieval Customs of Cluny*, edited by Susan Boynton and Isabelle Cochelin (Turnhout, 2005), 221-50.

[64] Clayton, *The Cult of the Virgin Mary*, 67-68. Jean Leclercq has dated the manuscript in which it is found (London: British Library, MS Cotton Titus D. xxvii), to 1012-1020, although he concedes the office may be earlier. Jean Leclercq, 'Formes anciennes de l'office marial', *Ephemerides Liturgicae*, 74 (1960), 89-102. See Roper, *Medieval English Benedictine Liturgy*, 219 for a transcription.

[65] See Dewick, *Facsimiles of 'Horae de beata Maria virgine'*, xvii, xiii-xiv for a general discussion.

various monastic rules, including the *Regularis Concordia*, in a manuscript from Christ Church, Canterbury, copied *circa* 1050.⁶⁶ It shares numerous similarities with an office found at the beginning of a Psalter from Nunnaminster, the female religious house associated with Winchester: although the manuscript dates from 1066-1087, it likely represents Anglo-Saxon usage.⁶⁷ Both the Christ Church and Nunnaminster offices are noticeably different from later continental sources, particularly in the texts used for the lessons of Matins, pointing to a separate development of the Hours of the Virgin on either side of the Channel.⁶⁸ The fact that these offices were performed together by the community is suggested, in the case of the Nunnaminster example, by the presence of a prayer preceding the text of the office itself. The prayer asks for Mary to inflict punishment on those who have despoiled the convent of its lands following the Conquest.⁶⁹ Not only does this add a crucial historical dimension to the significance of the Little Office, it points to a communal practice whose aim was to secure the protection of the community performing it on a daily basis.⁷⁰

Despite the evidence that the Little Office was communally-performed in the eleventh century, in the early-twelfth it seems once again to have reflected a particularly special, individual devotion to the Virgin. It does not appear in the monastic Constitutions drawn up by Lanfranc (d. 1089), the first post-Conquest archbishop of Canterbury instated by William I.⁷¹ It

---

⁶⁶ London: British Library, MS Cotton Tiberius A. iii. See Roper, *Medieval English Benedictine Liturgy*, 69.

⁶⁷ London: British Library, MS Royal 2. B. v. Roper, *Medieval English Benedictine Liturgy*, 71. Dewick described the similarities in his edition, Dewick, *Facsimiles of 'Horae de beata Maria virgine'*, xiv-xix.

⁶⁸ The continental examples almost universally feature a pseudo-Augustinian sermon for the feast of the Assumption as the readings for the lessons of Matins, while the English sources have texts from the *Song of Songs*. See Dewick, *Facsimiles of 'Horae de beata Maria virgine'*, columns 20-21, 4-5, and commentary, xviii.

⁶⁹ For a transcription and description of the text, see Clayton, *The Cult of the Virgin Mary*, 74-75.

⁷⁰ Clayton, *The Cult of the Virgin Mary*, 74, and Dewick, *Facsimiles of 'Horae de beata Maria virgine'*, xii.

⁷¹ Lanfranc's Constitutions nevertheless maintained the Hours for the Trinity and for the dead. See *The Monastic Constitutions of Lanfranc*, edited by

nevertheless continued to function as a marker of personal piety. William of Malmesbury's *Life* of Bishop Wulfstan of Worcester (d. 1095) mentions the saint taking a monk as company in his all-night vigils, which included the Little Office. [72] The chronicle of John of Worcester describes two further individuals whose personal love for Mary was demonstrated through the performance of the Little Office, among other practices: 'This servant of God [Benedict, Abbot of Tewkesbury Abbey (d. 1137)] was completely devoted to the most blessed and glorious Mother of God. Chanting the hours every day, he would either celebrate on a festival or hear a Mass in her honour. We know that the lord prior of Worcester [Warin (d. 1142)] does likewise'.[73] Their behaviour may have paved the way for Geoffrey of Gorron (d. 1146), Abbot of St Albans, and his successor Ralph (d. 1151), to make the Little Office a communal practice at the abbey.[74] Anselm of Bury St Edmunds is credited in the Bury Customary with doing the same.[75] From her review of the liturgical evidence, Sally Roper concludes that, 'communal daily recitation of all or part of this office [the Little Office] seems to have been commonplace in English Benedictine houses by *circa* 1250'.[76] There may be no concrete indication that the Little Office was deliberately downgraded from the public to private sphere after the Conquest – although Lanfranc was not adverse to reforming liturgical custom – but it was clearly once

---

Christopher N. L. Brooke and David Knowles (Oxford, 2002). For a discussion, see Roper, *Medieval English Benedictine Liturgy*, 43-44 and 69.

[72] William of Malmesbury, *Saints' Lives*, edited by Michael Winterbottom and Rodney M. Thomson (Oxford, 2002), 111-13.

[73] John of Worcester, *The Chronicle of John of Worcester*, edited and translated by Reginald R. Darlington and Patrick McGurk (Oxford, 1995), 223-25.

[74] A breviary from the abbacy of Geoffrey (London: British Library, MS Royal 2 A. x), contains a three-nocturn commemorative Marian office. Another Little Office is found in an ordinal from Wherwall based on a St Albans Psalter from the abbacy of Ralph, now Cambridge: Jesus College, MS C. 18 and London: British Library, MS Additional 21927.

[75] Et cotidie unam missam de ea, et post canonicas horas alias in honore eius celebrandas decrevit. *The Customary of the Benedictine Abbey of Bury St Edmunds in Suffolk*, edited and translated by Antonia Gransden (London, 1973), 122.

[76] Roper, *Medieval English Benedictine Liturgy*, 57.

more gaining traction as a public practice when the first miracle collections were composed.⁷⁷

Feast Days: Aelfsige and the Conception Debate

The desire to promote unique or especially elaborate practices of Marian devotion in the early part of the twelfth century is further supported by stories describing the miraculous foundation of feast days commemorating important events in Mary's life. Some of these feasts were well established. Dominic of Evesham describes the first celebration of the feast of Mary's Nativity, in which an extremely humble and virtuous man annually hears celestial singing (*caelestem harmoniam*) on the eve of the feast. When an angel reveals what the music is celebrating, he promptly institutes the official feast day.⁷⁸ According to William of Malmesbury, the eleventh-century bishop Fulbert of Chartres is thought to have enthusiastically endorsed the same feast, producing a number of sermons and responsories for it; William goes on to say that he does not need to enumerate them, as they had become famous from having merited Fulbert three drops of Mary's milk.⁷⁹ William also includes a story about the foundation of the Purification by the Emperor Justinian (527-565) after his people were restored from

---

⁷⁷ The main evidence for Lanfranc's challenge to Anglo-Saxon traditions is from the Council of Winchester in 1072, on which see Dorothy Whitelock, Martin Brett and Christopher N. L. Brooke, *Councils and Synods with Other Documents Relating to the English Church, 871-1204* (Oxford, 1981), 597, 607, and Martin Brett, 'A collection of Anglo-Norman councils', *Journal of Ecclesiastical History*, 26 (1975), 301-08. Additional testimony is provided by Eadmer of Canterbury, *The Life of St Anselm, Archbishop of Canterbury*, translated by Richard W. Southern (Oxford, 1962), 49-51.

⁷⁸ Dominic of Evesham, *De miraculis*, 274.

⁷⁹ Posterioribus annis fuit in eadem urbe Fulbertus episcopus cuius industria et litterarum peritia praecipue in amore sanctae Mariae excelluit. Denique non contentus aeternae virginis ab antiquo celebratis sollemniis, suo potissimum curavit exemplo, ut nativitas eius toto coleretur orbe latino. Praeterea laudum adiecit cumulo sermonem et responsoria, quae per se satis nota, notas nostras non desiderant. William of Malmesbury, *De laudibus et miraculis*, 82. This attribution is also found in William of Malmesbury, *Gesta regum Anglorum: The History of the English Kings. Volume 1*, edited and translated by Roger A. B. Mynors, Rodney M. Thomson and Michael Winterbottom (Oxford, 1998), 518-19.

plagues by the procession of a Marian image around Rome.[80] Whether or not it was due to the enduring memory of such miracles, the feasts of Mary's Nativity and Purification became widespread features of liturgical calendars across Europe well before the stories were incorporated into the first collections.[81]

In addition to the standard Marian feasts, far less common feasts came to feature in miraculous accounts. One is a feast of Mary celebrated on 18 December in the Visigothic calendar. It was intended as an alternative to the Annunciation feast of March 25, since the latter often fell during Lent, thereby limiting the degree of pomp with which it could be celebrated. In order to properly honour Mary as the feast's subject, the celebration was moved to December by Hildefonsus, Bishop of Toledo (d. 667), who additionally wrote a treatise defending Mary's virginity pre- and post-partum.[82] In the *Life* written for him by one of his successors, Cixila (d. 783), Hildefonsus is said to have received the miraculous reward of a pallium from the Virgin herself in return for his promotion of the feast.[83] Extracted from the hagiography, this story became a permanent fixture in the Marian miracle collections, often coming first, as it had in the series attributed to Anselm of Bury. This is significant, because although the feast was by and large limited to the Iberian Peninsula, it makes an exceptional appearance in the Bury Customary and in an ordinance issued by Anselm of Bury as a feast he himself instated at the abbey.[84] A

---

[80] William of Malmesbury, *De laudibus et miraculis*, 168-70. The feast of the Purification was actually instated by Pope Sergius I (687-701). Éric Palazzo and Ann-Katrin Johansson, 'Jalons liturgiques pour une histoire du culte de la Vierge dans l'Occident latin (V\ :sup:`e`-XI\ :sup:`e` siècle)', in *Marie: le Culte de la Vierge dans la société médiévale*, edited by Dominique Iogna-Prat, Éric Palazzo and Daniel Russo (Paris, 1996), 15-43.

[81] For a brief history of Marian feasts, see Palazzo and Johansson, 'Jalons liturgiques', 15-19.

[82] Hildefonsus of Toledo, *La virginidad perpetua de Santa Maria*, edited and translated by Julio Campos Ruiz (Madrid, 1971).

[83] Athanasius Braegelmann, 'The Life and Writings of Saint Ildefonsus of Toledo', unpublished doctoral thesis (Catholic University of America, 1942), 24. See also Jaime Ferreiro Alemparte, 'Las versiones latinas de la leyenda de San Ildefonso y su reflejo en Berceo', *Boletín de la Real Academia Española*, 50 (1970), 205-68.

[84] Anselmus duas apud nos solemnitates instituit, scilicet conceptionem sancte Marie que iam in multis ecclesiis per ipsum celebriter observatur, et

calendar from the period of his abbacy identified as East Anglian in origin features this unique practice, giving liturgical evidence for its celebration.[85]

Another very unusual observance that first appeared in England at this time was the feast of Mary's mother Anne. While not strictly a foundation legend, a miracle appears in William of Malmesbury's collection that extends veneration of Mary to her mother. In the tale, Guy, the bishop of the Pyrenean city of Lescar, is taken prisoner by Muslims in a military attack, *circa* 1134. He prays to the Virgin for liberation, but she appears to him in a vision, urging him instead to address her mother: 'If you begged me for love of St Anne, my beloved mother, and by your fervent prayers attained her as intermediary for you with my only Son, you would be freed from your prison chains and more quickly obtain the grace of bodily freedom'.[86] Guy does so, and his ransom is paid the following day. The inclusion of Anne in an appeal to Mary is noteworthy because of the evidence that the wholly unprecedented feast of Anne was first celebrated in the 1130s at Worcester Cathedral, a Marian foundation with which William had close ties. A letter dated to 1138 from Osbert of Clare (d. *c*. 1158) to Simon, Bishop of Worcester (d. 1150), responds to the Bishop's request for a series of texts for the liturgical celebration of the feast of Anne, all of which follow the letter in the manuscript.[87] Simon had apparently told

---

commemorationem eius in adventu quam Hildefonsus episcopus instituit. Gransden, *The customary of the Benedictine Abbey of Bury St. Edmunds*, 122 and 96-99. See also Gransden, 'The Cult of St Mary at Beodricisworth', 648-49.

[85] London: British Library, MS Cotton Cleopatra B. iii. Cf. Gransden, 'The Cult of St Mary at Beodricisworth', 647, note 100.

[86] Si exorares me, pro amore sanctae Annae, dilectae genitricis meae, et praecordialibus votis, ipsam interventricem tibi adquireres apud unigenitum filium meum, a vinculis carceralibus solutus recederes, et libertatis corporeae gratiam citius obtineres. William of Malmesbury, *De miraculis*, 91. For the historical background of the text, see Baudouin de Gaiffier 'A propos de Guy, évêque de Lescar et du culte de Sainte Anne', *Analecta Bollandiana*, 88, 1-2 (1970), 74.

[87] The letter is Epistle 12, Osbert of Clare, *The Letters of Osbert of Clare*, edited by Edward W. Williamson (Oxford, 1929), 77-78. The liturgical texts are omitted from the edition, and are found together in London: British Library, MS Cotton Vitellius A. xvii, the manuscript of Osbert's collected letters. The hymns are nevertheless also found in *Analecta Hymnica* 15:186 and 33:36.

Osbert that the feast was already being observed with an octave and additional meals.[88] Evidence of its ongoing observance at Worcester comes in the form of a sequence from the second half of the twelfth century found in a Troper/Proser.[89] In addition, multiple litanies from this period, copied at Worcester, feature Anne as first among the virgins.[90] From Worcester the feast spread throughout England, as attested in liturgical manuscripts produced at Winchester, St Augustine's, Ely, Christ Church and Evesham.[91]

Interest in the feast of Anne in England was very likely sparked by the much debated and similarly unique English feast of Mary's Conception. Its history is worth going into some detail here, since it has been used to explain the very inception of the collections in England at this time and presents an intriguing case study of miraculous support for contentious liturgical practice. The feast, which honours Mary's Conception by her own mother Anne, is the subject of a popular foundation story with a revealing setting. Shortly after the Conquest, the abbot of St Augustine's Canterbury, Elsinus or Aelfsige, is said to have been sent by William the Conqueror on a diplomatic mission to the King of Denmark in order to prevent an invasion by the Danes of the newly conquered English territory. After a successful mission, Aelfsige returns by ship to England but a storm threatens his passage. He and the rest of the crew pray, at which point a ghostly figure appears. The apparition, dressed as a bishop, instructs Aelfsige that if he is to reach land safely, he must first promise to observe the feast that honours Mary's Conception. Aelfsige naturally does so, and he and his crew

---

[88] Ep. 12, Osbert of Clare, *Letters*, 77.

[89] London: British Library, MS Cotton Caligula A. xiv, ff. 71v-72v. It is edited in *Analecta Hymnica* 34:55-56.

[90] For example, Cambridge: Corpus Christi College, 391, and Oxford: Magdalene College, 100, on which see Richard Pfaff, *The Liturgy in Medieval England: A History* (Cambridge, 2009), 213-14.

[91] These are: London: British Library, MS Cotton Vit. E. xviii (Winchester calendar); Oxford: Bodleian Library, Ashmole MS 1525 (St Augustine's calendar); Cambridge: Corpus Christi College, 270 (St Augustine's missal), Cambridge University Library MS Ii.4.20 (Ely missal); London: British Library, MS Cotton Tib. B. iii (Christ Church calendar); Oxford: Bodleian Library, Auct. MS D. 4. 6, f. 247^v (Reading litany), London: British Library, Add. MS 44874 (Evesham litany), and Oxford: Bodleian Library, Barlow MS 41 (Evesham litany).

are saved, upon which he performs the task he swore he would undertake, making the feast known far and wide.

It has been pointed out that the account is based on historical fact.[92] There was an abbot of St Augustine's and later of Ramsey named Aelfsige. He made his way to Denmark sometime in the 1080s, although this was most likely due to his being exiled on account of his closeness with the disgraced Anglo-Saxon archbishop Stigand and not because he was favoured by William I as a useful diplomat.[93] Rather than assume the redactor was ignorant of this fact, however, it makes more sense to see the story as an attempt to lend authority to the account by portraying the renegade cleric as close to the royal establishment.[94] The reason why this would have been important has much to do with the liturgical content of the story. The dialogue between the ghostly bishop and Aelfsige is noteworthy:

> 'If you wish to escape from the danger of the sea, if you wish to return to your native country safely, promise me in the presence of God that you will solemnly celebrate and observe the feast day of the conception of the mother of Christ'. Then the abbot said: 'How am I to do this or on what day?' The messenger said: 'You will celebrate it on the eighth day of December and will preach wherever you can, that it may be celebrated by everybody'. Elsinus said: 'And what sort of divine service do you command us to use on this feast?' He replied to him: 'Let every service which is said at her nativity be said also at her conception. Thus, when her birthday is mentioned at her nativity, let her conception be mentioned in this other celebration'. After the abbot heard this, he reached the English shore with a favourable wind blowing. Soon he made known everything he had seen or heard to whomever he could, and he ordered in the church at Ramsey, over

---

[92] See Marielle Lamy, *L'Immaculée Conception: étapes et enjeux d'une controverse au moyen-âge (XIIe-XVe siècles)* (Paris, 2000), 91, and Southern, 'The English origins', 196.

[93] On English clerics exiled or escaped to Denmark after the Conquest, see Erik Niblaeus, 'German Influence on Religious Practice in Scandinavia, *c.* 1050-1150', unpublished doctoral thesis, (University of London, King's College, 2010), 157-60.

[94] Southern argued that its author badly confused the historical information he had received. Southern, 'The English origins', 196.

which he had presided, that this feast be solemnly celebrated on 8 December.[95]

The level of detail in this story is striking. The precision with which the abbot is instructed about when and how the feast of the Conception is to be celebrated suggests a desire to teach the tale's readers and listeners.[96] The account's didactic quality would therefore corroborate the narrative of a feast that was largely unknown and was only beginning to spread in the post-Conquest period, helped along by the familiarity and status of its legendary founder.

The Aelfsige legend would have us believe that the Conception feast saw its first appearance at the abbey of Ramsey some time in the late eleventh century. It was nevertheless being celebrated some fifty years earlier in the major cathedrals of the Anglo-Saxon kingdom. Originally a Byzantine feast, the Conception had been adopted in England following the tenth-century reform movement, possibly due to Byzantine monks coming to England via Southern Italy.[97] Mention of the feast, as well as liturgical texts for its celebration, are found in several manuscripts dated between 1032 and 1065 from Christ Church Canterbury, Worcester, Winchester and Exeter.[98] It remained a unique English practice, celebrated nowhere else in Europe apart from isolated Italian houses subject to Greek influence, such as the monastery of St Saba in Rome, populated by monks fleeing the iconoclast controversy in the eighth

---

[95] Translated by Clayton, *The Cult of the Virgin Mary*, 48-49.

[96] The version that appears in a mid-twelfth-century collection is notably pro-Norman. *Liber de miraculis Sanctae Dei genitricis Mariae*, edited by Thomas Crane (Ithaca, 1925), 22.

[97] Clayton, *The Cult of the Virgin Mary*, 44.

[98] Calendars found in London: British Library, MS Cotton Vitellius E. xviii and in London: British Library, MS Cotton Titus D. xxvii are both from Winchester and date from *circa* 1030 to 1057. Cambridge: Corpus Christi College, MS 391, another calendar from Worcester, dates from *circa* 1065. London: British Library, MS Harley 2892; Le Havre: Bibliothèque Municipale, MS 330, and Oxford: Bodleian Library, Bodl. MS 579, from the first half of the eleventh century contain liturgical texts from Christ Church, Exeter and Winchester. On these see Clayton, *The Cult of the Virgin Mary*, 44-46.

century. Notably, Anselm of Bury had himself been abbot of St Saba before taking up his post in England.[99]

A change is noticeable in the liturgical record by 1100 when the feast seems to have disappeared.[100] Edmund Bishop argued that this 'eclipse' was no accident, but rather the result of a purposeful removal.[101] His argument drew from a treatise composed *circa* 1125 by Eadmer of Christ Church Canterbury, which places the blame for the feast's disappearance squarely, if not explicitly, on sceptical newcomers such as Lanfranc.[102] Eadmer writes:

> I wish to consider today's celebration, by which the conception of Mary, blessed mother of God has been restored as a feast day in many places ... it was celebrated more frequently in ancient times, especially in those times in which simplicity and a more humble devotion to God flourished. Where greater learning and knowledge imbued and raised up the minds of certain men, it made them remove that same celebration from the public eye in scorn of the simplicity of poor men, and reduced it to nothing, as if it lacked all justification. Their decision to be rid of it was made with great zeal, because they, who made the decision, were pre-eminent in the abundance of both their secular and ecclesiastical authority and in their wealth ... they did not fear to abolish the feast, that is to say of the conception of the most

---

[99] Clayton, *The Cult of the Virgin Mary*, 44.

[100] None of the post-Conquest calendars from the cathedrals mentioned above contain the feast, as has been recognized by Thomas A. Heslop, 'The Canterbury calendars and the Norman Conquest', in *Canterbury and the Norman Conquest: Churches, Saints and Scholars 1066-1109*, edited by Richard Eales and Richard Sharpe (London, 1995), 53-62, and Richard W. Pfaff, 'Lanfranc's supposed purge of the Anglo-Saxon Calendar', in *Warriors and Churchmen in the High Middle Ages: Essays Presented to Karl Leyser*, edited by Timothy Reuter (London, 1992), 104.

[101] Edmund Bishop, 'On the Origins of the Feast of the Conception of the Blessed Virgin Mary', in *Liturgica Historica: Papers on the Liturgy and Religious Life of the Western Church* (Oxford, 1918), 249.

[102] Most scholars have taken this as fact, i.e. Jean Fournée, 'Du *De conceptu virginali* de Saint Anselm au *De conceptione Sanctae Mariae* de son disciple Eadmer: ou de *la Virgo purissima* à *la Virgo immaculata*', in *Les mutations socio-culturelles au tournant des XIe-XIIe siècles*, edited by Raymonde Foreville (Paris, 1984), 713, and Jay Rubenstein, 'Liturgy against history: the competing visions of Lanfranc and Eadmer', *Speculum*, 74 (1999), 305. While contesting Lanfranc's willful alteration of the Anglo-Saxon liturgy, Richard Pfaff accepts the feast's disappearance in Pfaff, 'Lanfranc's supposed purge', 95-108.

sacred lady, by the reason of their authority and the wisdom of their souls, by which they boasted that they could prevail.[103]

The rest of the treatise presents Eadmer's arguments in favour of taking up the feast once more, which amounts to the first ever articulation of the doctrine of Mary's Immaculate Conception.[104] This radical new doctrine claimed that Mary had been exempt from original sin at her conception. It resulted therefore from one monk's attempt to defend a liturgical celebration by giving it the strongest theological justification he could: if Mary's conception were utterly unique, how could it not be commemorated?

Eadmer was not alone in showing interest in the feast of the Conception. A letter written by Osbert of Clare in 1128 indicates that it was of pressing concern for a number of prominent English clerics. Addressing Anselm of Bury St Edmunds, Osbert asked that the abbot support a bid to reinstate the feast, following an altercation at Westminster in which Roger, Bishop of Salisbury (d. 1139) and Bernard, Bishop of St David's (d. 1148), cancelled the celebration as it was underway.[105] Osbert sought Anselm's advice on how to answer these men and all those who argued that the feast lacked the necessary authority. He approached Anselm mainly because the abbot was known to have instated the feast at Bury 'and

---

[103] Mihi considerare volenti occurrit hodierna solemnitas, quae de conceptione beatae Matris Dei Mariae multis in locis festiva recolitur. Et quidem priscis temporibus frequentiori usu celebrabatur, ab iis praecipue in quibus pura simplicitas et humilior in Deum vigebat devotio. At ubi et major scientia et praepollens examinatio rerum mentes quorumdam imbuit et erexit, eamdem solemnitatem, spreta pauperum simplicitate, de medio sustulit; et eam quasi ratione vacantem redegit in nihil. Quorum sententia eo maxime in robur excrevit quod ii, qui eam protulerunt, saeculari et ecclesiastica auctoritate divitiarumque abundantia praeeminebant ... festum scilicet de conceptione ipsius sacratissimae dominae sua qua se pollere gloriabantur auctoritatis ratione abolere non timuerunt. Eadmer of Canterbury, *Tractatus de conceptione beatae Mariae*, edited by Herbert Thurston and Thomas Slater (Freiburg, 1904), 1, 5.

[104] There have not been many studies that deal with this treatise and none in any great detail. A. W. Burridge provides a schematic outline, along with questions of dating, in A. W. Burridge, 'L'Immaculée Conception dans la théologie de l'Angleterre médiévale', *Revue d'Histoire Ecclésiastique*, 32 (1936), 570-97. Marielle Lamy discusses the treatise only sporadically, and not at any length, in her book. Lamy, *L'Immaculée Conception*, 34-35, 118-19.

[105] These were Roger, Bishop of Salisbury, and Bernard, Bishop of St Davids.

it is by your persistency that the feast of her Conception is celebrated in many places', continued Osbert.[106] Osbert also encouraged Anselm to enlist the aid of other supporters, including the bishop of London and abbot of Reading.[107] The matter was ultimately decided in favour of the feast's official reinstatement at the Council of London of 1129, presided over by Henry I and a papal legate.[108] The case of the Conception feast illustrates how what to us might seem a marginal quibble over an obscure liturgical practice was in fact a hotly contested issue in its day.

Due to the polemical nature of the English history of the feast of Mary's Conception, Edmund Bishop argued that the story of Aelfsige was created as part of the dossier with which the feast's advocates lent support to their case. A miraculous origin for the feast would have greatly strengthened claims for its celebration, and more so if it were a very recent miracle set in a familiar location involving an individual favoured by the king himself. But scholars

---

[106] Osbert of Clare, *Letters*, 65. Evidence of Anselm's adoption of the feast at Bury is found in Charter 112, David C. Douglas, *Feudal Documents from the Abbey of Bury St Edmunds* (Oxford, 1932), 112-13, and *Customary of the Benedictine Abbey of Bury St Edmunds*, 96-99. On this, see Gransden, 'The cult of St Mary', 648-49.

[107] These were Gilbert, so-called the Universal, Bishop of London, and Hugh, Abbot of Reading. On Gilbert, see Gilbert the Universal, *Glossa ordinaria in lamentationes Ieremie prophete*, edited by Alexander Andrée, Studia Latina Stockholmiensia, 52 (Stockholm, 2005), 37-40. On Hugh of Reading, see Jean Fournée, 'La place de Rouen et de la Normandie dans le développement du culte et de l'iconographie de l'Immaculée-Conception', in *Histoire religieuse de la Normandie*, edited by Guy-Marie Oury (Chambray, 1981), 125, 129 and 131.

[108] Although not in the record of the council itself, the decision is recorded in the *Annales de Theokesberia, 1066-1263*, edited by Henry Richards Luard, *Annales Monastici*, volume 1, Rolls Series, 36 (London, 1864), 45. Darlington and McGurk indicated the shared similarities of this entry with that of the Worcester Chronicle: John of Worcester, *Chronicle*, 188. Paul Hayward's recent edition of the Winchcombe Chronicle, as a witness to John of Worcester's, points to the fact that this particular entry derives from a Gloucester source. *The Winchcombe and Coventry Chronicles: Hitherto Unnoticed Witnesses to the Work of John of Worcester*, edited and translated by Paul Antony Hayward (Tempe, Arizona, 2010), 115-16. Other monastic houses record their adoption of the feast around the date of the council, for example St Peter's, Gloucester, *Historia et cartularium monasterii Sancti Petri Gloucestriae*, edited by William Henry Hart, Rolls Series, 33 (London, 1863), 15, and Winchcombe, London: British Library, MS Cotton Tiberius E. iv.

have since gone on to extend the argument to include the miracle collections more generally.[109] The fact that Anselm of Bury was involved in the dispute over the feast and is also credited with having commissioned or redacted one of the first collections presents convincing proof of their role in bolstering the re-adoption of the feast. Yet this ignores the fact that the Aelfsige legend does not appear in the earliest manuscripts of the collections, which probably predated the Conception controversy.[110] The collections clearly did not originate, therefore, solely for the purpose of advocating for the reinstatement of the Conception feast.

Analysis of the Aelfsige legend suggests we must widen our understanding of what motivated the first compilers of the Marian miracle collections. Their interest did not lie exclusively in supporting the feast of the Conception, but in supporting a much broader range of liturgical commemorations. The diverse forms of liturgical practice present in the miracles suggest a concern with the development of the Marian cult in its many varied expressions. Miraculous support would have been all the more essential in the case of practices that were in the process of being developed and spreading, such as the Little Office. Controversy over increasingly elaborate forms of venerating the Virgin, particularly if they hearkened back to what may have been regarded as outmoded or peculiar Anglo-Saxon tradition, would explain the need to circulate miraculous accounts of the rewards such practices could garner those who performed them. It is therefore hardly a coincidence that the earliest Marian miracles were compiled at institutions where such unique liturgical practices were being adopted: Bury St Edmunds, Malmesbury, Evesham; although liturgical sources from twelfth-century Malmesbury and Evesham do not survive, those from other institutions with important links to both houses certainly signal the embrace of novel liturgies. The collections can therefore be understood as compendia of proper commemorative

---

[109] Bishop, 'Origins', 249. See also Southern, 'The English origins', 194, and most recently, Adrienne Williams Boyarin, *Miracles of the Virgin in Medieval England: Law and Jewishness in Marian Legends* (Cambridge, 2010), 20.

[110] These are found in London: Lambeth Palace Library, MS 214 and Rome: Vatican Lib., Reg. Lat. MS 543.

practice: advertising the good that comes of celebrating Mary's sanctity in the widest possible variety of forms, both old and new.

Thus far, we have seen how miracles could act as useful apologetic texts for the adoption and continuation of liturgical practices that were novel or the subject of debate. Their efficacy in supporting these devotions is further attested by their incorporation into the very liturgies they were recorded to champion. A notable example of this process is found in a twelfth-century *libellum* containing a collection of Marian miracle stories that is attached to and in the same hand as an office for the feast of the Conception from Saint-Martin-des-Champs.[111] It is possible that the abbey, reformed under the influence of Cluny in 1079, received both the office and the miracle collection together from England, perhaps from Reading, another Cluniac-reformed institution, founded in 1121, whose first abbot, Hugh, instated the Conception feast at the abbey and is known to have had ties to Saint-Martin-des-Champs.[112] The office in the Saint-Martin-des-Champs manuscript has considerable similarities with a thirteenth-century office for the feast in an Ely manuscript, supporting the idea of an English source for both.[113]

The Aelfsige legend is among the miracles in the Saint-Martin collection, and may later have made its way into the liturgy for the feast day; Solange Corbin has traced the gradual adoption of the story, as the main readings for the monastic office of Matins for the feast day, to no later than the thirteenth century.[114] A legendary

[111] Paris: Bibliothèque Nationale, MS Lat. 18168. For the history of Saint-Martin-des-Champs, see Paul Huguet, *Notice historique sur l'ancien prieuré Saint-Martin-des-Champs et sur le conservatoire impérial des arts et métiers* (Neuilly, 1859), 4-5.

[112] Hugh wrote a Marian prayer for a fellow monk at Saint-Martin-des-Champs. Jean Fournée, 'La place de Rouen et de la Normandie dans le développement du culte et de l'iconographie de l'Immaculée-Conception', in *Histoire religieuse de la Normandie*, edited by Guy-Marie Oury (Chambray, 1981), 131, also 125, 129, and Denis Hüe, 'La fête normande', in *Provinces, Régions, Terroirs au Moyen Age de la Réalité à l'Imaginaire*, edited by Bernard Guidot (Strasbourg, 1991), 41-42.

[113] Osbert of Clare wrote in 1128 that the feast was adopted by Hugh, Abbot of Reading, at the behest of Henry I himself. Osbert of Clare, *Letters*, 67.

[114] Solange Corbin lists ten thirteenth-century manuscripts, from both sides of the Channel, that contain the Aelfsige legend as readings for the office of Matins, though none before this period. Solange Corbin, '*Miracula beatae*

from the Parisian abbey of Saint-Germain-des-Près gives us a clear indication of how miracles were incorporated into the liturgies of feast days as early as the twelfth century. It contains a collection of miracles, among which is the Aelfsige legend, as readings for the *collatio* (a short reading before Compline) and for *prandium* (dinner) on the feast day of the Conception.[115] This evidence points to the inextricable connection between miracles and liturgy.

Miracles did not simply provide additional textual support underpinning novel liturgical practices, but were themselves incorporated as performative elements in these very same practices. We might see this as creating a positive feedback loop, justifying a particular practice with every retelling of the miracles it came to include. Ritually promoting the liturgy with each recitation, miracles were therefore instrumental to the liturgy's preservation, reaffirming for the monks and nuns who sang Mary's praises in antiphon, Mass and office that she was indeed worthy of this celebration, and would perhaps even bestow the same rewards on them in return for their commemoration of her past acts of mercy.

Conclusion

Marian miracles eventually became one of the most popular forms of devotional literature in medieval Europe, yet their initial appearance and early development must be situated in the context of Anglo-Norman monastic culture. The origins of Marian miracle collections is explained in great part by the prolific production of hagiographical materials designed to fix and promote the cult of saints in a time of upheaval, as English monks took it upon themselves to do for her what they were doing for other Anglo-Saxon saints. The literary context alone does not, however, provide us with the ultimate reason for the appearance of collections of Marian miracles. We cannot forget that the cult of saints had a strongly performative element that included pilgrimage and the veneration of relics, yet the cult of the Virgin could not be conceived of in the same way, in the absence of a body to venerate.

Mariae semper virginis', in *Cahiers de Civilisation Médiévale*, 39-40 (1967), 420.

[115] Paris: Bibliothèque Nationale, MS lat. 12606, fol. 171v.

The miracles compiled by Anglo-Norman monks therefore privileged a different sort of action that garnered Mary's miraculous intervention. The liturgical practices surveyed here, the Hail Mary, antiphons and responsories, Masses and full Offices in addition to the celebration of feast days, are depicted as the principal ways to obtain Mary's favour. More often than not, these are shown to be the domain primarily of religious professionals, reinforcing the idea that the miracles were the product of a monastic context – written by monks, for monks – at least at this early date. Liturgical practice was of special importance for monks whose lives were significantly occupied with its performance. It was more relevant still for those monks who were charged with recording and preserving the history of their abbeys, including the lives of their saints: William, Dominic and Anselm were all extremely active in writing or commissioning histories and hagiographies, the latter of which were integral to the celebration of liturgical feasts. In recording Mary's miraculous actions, they were in fact building a history for the liturgical traditions of their institutions, justifying Mary's centrality for each institution's identity, past and present.

The importance of the liturgy in the Marian cult and the place of the cult in English Benedictine houses provides crucial background for understanding why the liturgy features so heavily in the earliest miracle collections. This was particularly the case when the practice in question was subject to reform and alteration, as were the feast of the Conception and possibly the Little Office, following the Norman Conquest. When understood as a central element of the corporate, monastic identities of English institutions, an essential part of their heritage, it is little wonder that any diminution of Marian liturgies could become a source of controversy, one in which miracle accounts had a key role to play. Incorporated into liturgical ritual as readings at Matins, *collatio* and at meal times, miracles provided miraculous justification for that ritual's very existence. But while the liturgical practices discussed here were adopted or developed to an unusual degree in Anglo-Norman England, they were not limited by geography. It was not necessary for a church or abbey to be dedicated to the Virgin to celebrate Marian Masses, offices and feast days. This ultimately allowed the kinds of liturgical practice featured in the miracle stories to spread throughout western Europe in the twelfth century, and the miracle collections with them. Marian miracles in collections copied and circulated on the example of the first English ones became integral to the rise and spread of the Marian cult as she emerged as the foremost saint in medieval Europe, promising rewards to any and all who would venerate her in increasingly diverse and elaborate ways.

CONCEPTIONS OF THE MIRACULOUS: NATURAL PHILOSOPHY AND MEDICAL KNOWLEDGE IN THE THIRTEENTH-CENTURY *MIRACULA* OF ST EDMUND OF ABINGDON

Louise Elizabeth Wilson

Therefore, this woman is twice presented for the inspection of the apostolic seat, and strictly examined by the cardinals, by the Lord Pope himself and by his physicians, and they touched, with fitting reverence, the place where the hump had been. In the end, faith furnishes everything, because she is restored to health by no work of nature.[1]

The authors of the thirteenth-century miracle collections of St Edmund of Abingdon (d. 1240) make frequent allusions to nature, physicians and medicine in their narratives. This is articulated succinctly in the above account, composed by Archbishop Albert of Armagh (d. 1273). Here, the Archbishop establishes a clear distinction between a miraculous cure, supplied by the woman's faith, and a cure effected by natural means, situating the concept of a miracle within broader discourses about the processes and operations governing the natural world.

The miracles of St Edmund were composed during a crucial period in the development of the concept of nature in western Christendom. The twelfth and thirteenth centuries experienced sweeping cultural and intellectual change, dramatically altering clerical perceptions of the natural and supernatural worlds. This

---

[1] Hec itaque mulier bis sedis apostolice conspectui est exhibita, et tam a cardinalibus quam ab ipso domino papa et ejus medicis strictissime examinata, et ea qua decuit reverentia in loco ubi gibbus insederat attrectata. Fidem in fine dedit omnibus quod non opus nature eam sanitati restituit: Auxerre: Bibliothèque Municipale d'Auxerre, Manuscrit 123G, fols 106vb-107ra.

was driven by access to translations of recently acquired Ancient Greek and Islamic medical and natural philosophical texts, which were distributed throughout the monasteries, cathedral schools and universities of Europe.[2] In particular, the rediscovery of the natural works of Aristotle led to a revised understanding of the physical world and a sharpening of the conceptual boundaries between the natural and supernatural.[3] These intellectual changes were not confined to university precincts and the cloistered corridors of the cathedral schools, but impinged on and altered the medieval clergy's approach to the supernatural, the sacred and the miraculous.

Historical investigation into the medieval concept of a miracle has detailed the influence of these ideas on high-level philosophical and theological notions of the miraculous, examining the writings and thought of elite scholars and theologians from Augustine to Aquinas.[4] An alternative approach, expounded in the work of Benedicta Ward and, more recently, Michael Goodich, lead us away from stratospherically academic considerations to explore the formulation of ideas about the miraculous expressed in hagiographical texts, revealing attitudes about the concept of a

[2] Vivian Nutton, 'Medicine in medieval western Europe, 1000-1500', in *The Western Medical Tradition 800 BC to AD 1800*, edited by Lawrence I. Conrad et al. (Cambridge, 1995), 139-206. Jean Jolivet, 'The Arabic inheritance', in *A History of Twelfth-Century Western Philosophy*, edited by Peter Dronke (Cambridge, 1988), 113-48.

[3] Marie-Dominique Chenu, *Nature, Man and Society in the Twelfth Century* (Chicago and London 1968); Roger French and Andrew Cunningham, *Before Science: The Invention of the Friar's Natural Philosophy* (Aldershot, 1996); Edward Grant, *The Foundations of Modern Science in the Middle Ages: Their Religious, Institutional and Intellectual Contexts* (Cambridge, 1996), 26-53. Lorraine Daston and Katharine Park, *Wonders and the Order of Nature, 1150-1750* (New York, 2001); Robert Bartlett, *The Natural and the Supernatural in the Middle Ages* (Cambridge, 2008).

[4] Joan Cadden, 'Science and rhetoric in the middle age: the natural philosophy of William of Conches', *Journal of the History of Ideas*, 56 (1995), 1-24. Michael E. Goodich, 'A chapter in the history of the Christian theology of miracle: Engelbert of Admont's (ca. 1250-1331) *Expositio super psalmum* 118 and *De miraculis Christi*', in *Cross Cultural Convergences in the Crusader Period*, edited by Michael E. Goodich, Sophia Menache and Sylvia Schein (New York, 1995), 89-110. John A. Hardon, 'The concept of miracle from St Augustine to modern apologetics', *Theological Studies*, 15 (1954), 229-57.

miracle prevalent in wider social, cultural and theological settings.[5] Similarly, in her examination of the fifteenth-century canonization records of Vincent Ferrer, Laura Smoller explored the relationship between learned and unlearned definitions of nature and miracle.[6] Scholarly interest in these broader definitions of the natural and supernatural has also focussed on the writings of twelfth and thirteenth-century chroniclers, investigating their authors' interpretation of wonders, marvels and miracles.[7]

In the context of this burgeoning interest in medieval ideas about the natural and supernatural worlds, the current chapter will assess the definition of a miracle articulated by the authors of two thirteenth-century *Miracula*, which document the miracles of St Edmund of Abingdon. Scrutiny of these specific texts provides a dissection of the thought of men familiar with this new learning, yet who were by no means at its speculative cutting edge. Examination of the definition of the miraculous presented in these accounts, reveals the ways in which their authors utilised newly emerging natural philosophical concepts, along with medical knowledge and the opinions of physicians, to validate their claims for a miracle. Our authors also drew from a personal experience with the natural world, a practical awareness of the typical observable processes inherent in nature. Detailed examination of the miracles of St Edmund reveals how practical knowledge, natural philosophy, medical theory and theology interacted to produce a

---

[5] Benedicta Ward, *Miracles and the Medieval Mind: Theory, Record and Event, 1000-1215*, 2nd edn (Aldershot, 1987). Michael E. Goodich, *Miracles and Wonders: the Development of the Concept of Miracle, 1150-1350* (Aldershot, 2007). Also see Caroline Walker Bynum, 'Miracles and marvels: the limits of alterity', in *Vita Religiosa im Mittelalter: Festschrift für Kaspar Elm zum 70. Geburtstag*, edited by Franz J. Felten and Nikolas Jaspert (Berlin, 1999), 799-817.

[6] Laura Smoller, 'Defining the boundaries of the natural in the fifteenth century: the inquest into the miracles of St. Vincent Ferrer (d. 1419)', *Viator*, 28 (1997), 333-59.

[7] Elizabeth Freeman, 'Wonders, prodigies and marvels: unusual bodies and the fear of heresy in Ralph of Coggeshall's *Chronicon Anglicanum*', *Journal of Medieval History*, 26 (2000), 127-43. Carl Watkins, 'Fascination and anxiety in medieval wonder stories', in *The Unorthodox Imagination in Late Medieval Britain*, edited by Sophie Page (Manchester, 2011), 45-64.

definition of a healing miracle which was conceptually distinct from the natural world.

Before considering this definition in much greater detail it is necessary to briefly survey the origins and authorship of St Edmund's miracle collections, providing a chronological and geographical context for the texts.

The Miracles of St Edmund: Text and Context

The most complete manuscript account of St Edmund's miracles resides in Burgundy at the Public Library in Auxerre, Manuscript 123G.[8] The manuscript contains two collections of miracles dating from the mid to late thirteenth century and was most probably kept at Pontigny Abbey, the site of St Edmund's body and shrine. The first document contained in the manuscript, entitled *History of the Canonization of St Edmund*, was composed by Archbishop Albert of Armagh, who had been one of the papal commissioners at St Edmund's canonization enquiry.[9] The text comprises an account of the process of the enquiry, accompanied by transcripts of letters promoting Archbishop Edmund's sanctity, papal communications to those conducting the enquiry and a copy of the canonization bull. Archbishop Albert also included an account of the translation of St Edmund's body, along with a sermon composed by himself for this occasion. Of greater significance to our present concerns, the text also contains a hagiographical account of twenty miracles ascribed to St Edmund.[10]

The prologue to Albert's work provides us with some indication of the author's motivation for writing this document. Albert of Armagh declared his intention to 'gather the fragments' of the

---

[8] Auxerre 123G. Selections from the Auxerre manuscript were published during the eighteenth century. Edmond Martène and Ursin Durand, '*Vita beati Edmundi Cantuariensis archiepiscopi*', *Thesaurus novus anecdotorum*, volume 3 (Paris, 1717), cols 1751-1928. An abridged copy of the Auxerre accounts, dating to the second half of the thirteenth century, can be found in Oxford: Bodleian Library, Manuscript Fell 2, fols 1-44. Bruce C. Barker-Benfield, *St Augustine's Abbey, Canterbury*, volume 3, Corpus of Medieval Library Catalogues, 13 (London, 2008), 1744.

[9] Clifford H. Lawrence, *St Edmund of Abingdon: A Study in Hagiography and History* (Oxford, 1960), 15.

[10] Martène and Durand, cols 1882-1890. Auxerre 123G, fols 104va-112vb.

procedure so that they would not be wasted.¹¹ This inclination to provide documentation recording consecutive stages in the canonization process of a saint was not unique to St Edmund's inquisition. Similar records of documents associated with canonization proceedings have been identified for both St Gilbert of Sempringham (canonized in 1202) and St Hugh of Lincoln (canonized in 1220).¹² The incorporation of evidence drawn from the canonization enquiry into hagiographical compositions was believed by their authors to lend additional credence to their miracle accounts. Archbishop Albert attested to this by assuring his audience that 'we will admit no miracle that will not have been confirmed by the lawful deposition of the sworn witnesses in the presence of the highest pontiff and his brothers'.¹³ In the eyes of the Archbishop, the evidential standards insisted upon by the curia, along with the favourable decision of the pope to canonize St Edmund, authenticated his hagiographical accounts of St Edmund's miracles.

The annotation and modification of Albert of Armagh's text by successive readers offers some indication of its usage. The presence of stress marks above the letters a, o, e and i, which were typically adopted to assist an orator when reading aloud, suggests that this section of the manuscript was either intended, or modified after creation, for oral presentation.¹⁴ Additionally, Albert of Armagh's sermon on the translation of St Edmund, which begins on a new quire at folio 57r, was accompanied by marginal notations separating it into twelve *lectiones*.¹⁵ This division into distinct

---

[11] Martène and Durand, 1832.

[12] Raymonde Foreville and Gillian Keir, *The Book of St Gilbert* (Oxford, 1987), cviii.

[13] Quod non fuerit legitima testium juratorum depositione coram summo pontifice & confratribus ejus firmatum. Auxerre 123G, fols 105rb-va.

[14] For example, Auxerre 123G, fols 14v and 57r. Teresa Webber, 'Monastic and cathedral book collections in the late eleventh and twelfth centuries', in *The Cambridge History of Libraries in Britain and Ireland*, volume 1, edited by Elisabeth Leedham-Green and Teresa Webber (Cambridge, 2006), 120.

[15] The subdivision of hagiographical works into lessons can also be found in the *Life of St Dunstan*, which in its earliest form was separated into twelve *lectiones*. Baudouin de Gaiffier, 'L'Hagiographie et son public au XIe siècle', in *Miscellanea historica in honorem Leonis van der Essen* (Brussels and Paris, 1947), 141-42.

lessons indicates a liturgical function for at least this segment of the manuscript. Consideration of the function of hagiographical texts has revealed a broad spectrum of uses, stretching from private reading, to readings for conventual lectures in both refectory and chapter and as material for the office or feast of a particular saint.[16] Drawing on the palaeographical evidence, it can be hesitatingly conjectured that at least one section of the Auxerre manuscript served just this type of liturgical function, and consequently may have been located at the site of St Edmund's shrine in Pontigny, where his liturgy would be regularly celebrated.

Our second collection of St Edmund's miracles, which forms the second half of Auxerre Manuscript 123G, can be dated through palaeographical evidence to the last quarter of the thirteenth century. It contains an anonymous account of around two hundred and thirty miracles ascribed to St Edmund. A number of the accounts recorded towards the end of the collection were drawn directly from Albert of Armagh's *Miracula*, indicating a familiarity on the part of the author with the Archbishop's earlier text. Although the author of this work remains unknown, the use of the *punctus flexus* mark in this section of the manuscript suggests a Cistercian authorship, possibly indicating Pontigny Abbey as the place of production.[17] There is evidence of a flourishing *scriptorium* at Pontigny from the mid-twelfth century and catalogues of the medieval library record the presence of several hagiographical works relevant to Pontigny's history, including a *Miracula* of St Thomas Becket, who, like Archbishop Edmund, had resided at Pontigny Abbey.[18] The author, like Archbishop Albert, claimed to be writing

---

[16] Baudouin de Gaiffier, 'L'hagiographie et son Public', 142. Baudouin de Gaiffier, 'A propos des légendiers latins', *Analecta Bollandiana*, 97 (1979), 60.

[17] The *punctus flexus* mark functioned as a minor medial pause separating the phrases within a clause. Charles H. Talbot, 'Notes on the library at Pontigny', *Analecta sacris ordinis cisterciensis*, 10 (Rome, 1954), 106-68. My sincere thanks extend to Professor Teresa Webber for her palaeographical advice.

[18] Talbot 'Notes on the library', 107. Monique Peyrafort-Huin identified hagiographical works, including John of Salisbury's *Passio* of St Thomas Becket and Benedict of Peterborough's *Miracula* of St Thomas, among the Pontigny collection. Monique Peyrafort-Huin, *La bibliothèque médiévale de l'abbaye de Pontigny (XIIe-XIXe siècles): histoire, inventaires anciens, manuscrits*

in order to preserve a record of the events for posterity.[19] The composition of this *Miracula* perhaps fits into a broader late twelfth and thirteenth-century trend, which saw an increase in writings recording God's activities amongst His faithful, in the format of chronicles, records of wonders and a vast outpouring of hagiographical literature.[20]

Physical examination of the manuscript provides some indications of its function and later usage by consecutive generations into the fourteenth century. The text does not appear to have functioned as promotional material for St Edmund's cult, since it did not circulate widely and only one (incomplete) copy, formerly at St Augustine's Abbey at Canterbury, still survives.[21] Marginal notations accompany the text, highlighting passages considered to be of importance. These markings included the phrase '*nota bene*', along with the underlining of text and the marking of passages with sketches of pointing fingers.[22] There are several marginal comments in a cursive script differing from the main hands in which the document was written.[23] The presence of catchwords, written once again in a cursive script, mark the quire breaks in this section of the manuscript, which suggest that the manuscript was rebound sometime after it had been composed, possibly during the fourteenth century. Having established the monastic authorship and usage of these manuscripts, a detailed examination of the content of these texts will now be presented investigating the authors' conceptions of the natural and the miraculous.

(Paris, 2001), 95. Lawrence, *St Edmund of Abingdon*, 176-82. Frank Barlow, *Thomas Becket* (London, 1997), 124.

[19] Auxerre 123G, fol. 113ra.

[20] For more on the activities of twelfth-century chroniclers see Carl S. Watkins, *History and the Supernatural in Medieval England* (Cambridge, 2007); Gabrielle Spiegel, *The Past as Text: The Theory and Practice of Medieval Historiography* (Baltimore, 1997); Nancy F. Partner, *Serious Entertainments: The Writing of History in Twelfth-Century England* (Chicago, 1977).

[21] Oxford: Bodleian Library, MS Fell 2, fols 1-44.

[22] Auxerre 123G, fols 74v (nota bene), 53v and 89v (pointing fingers), 50v-51r (underlining).

[23] Auxerre 123G, fols 32v and 91ra.

Conceptions of Nature in the Miracles of St Edmund

St Edmund's miracle collections convey their authors' belief in the existence of a natural order inherent in the world. In his introduction to the miracle collection, Albert of Armagh declared that miracles were worked 'against the order of nature', articulating this inextricable link between the concepts of the natural and the miraculous in thirteenth-century theology.[24] The Archbishop even presumed that his audience shared his own conviction that a miracle could have no natural explanation. Albert anticipated and refuted potential criticism of St Edmund's thaumaturgic abilities, which were based on contentions that cured individuals had recovered by natural means. He declared that 'men should be found detracting from the miracles of the saints and assigning certain [events] to the benefit of nature'.[25] Establishing just what these benefits of nature were allows us to investigate our authors' understanding of the boundaries and limitations of the natural world.

The author of the longer *Miracula* frequently refers to the concept of nature in narratives describing miracles benefitting women in childbirth. The women assisting Maria in a lengthy labour saw the arm of her unborn child emerging first, 'against the method and order of nature'.[26] The women (*obstetrices*) attending the stricken mother were further stunned when the child was 'beginning to be born against the method of giving birth and the

---

[24] Contra nature ordinem. Auxerre 123G, fol. 105rb.

[25] Licet reperiantur homines sanctorum miraculis derogantes & quedam nature beneficio attribuentes. Auxerre 123G, fol. 109ra-rb.

[26] Contra modum & ordinem nature. Auxerre 123G, fol. 137vb. There is considerable debate among historians about the existence of midwives as a professional occupational group before the second half of the thirteenth century. The term '*obstetrix*', which can be translated simply as 'she who stands by', may refer to any woman in attendance at the birthing chamber. Monica Green, in her expansive study of the developing roles of female practitioners during the central and later middle ages, argued that midwifery skills were dispersed throughout the community prior to the second half of the thirteenth century. Monica Green, *Making Women's Medicine Masculine: The Rise of Male Authority in Pre-modern Gynaecology* (Oxford, 2008), 136. For an insightful review of recent research in this area see Monica Green, 'Bodies, gender, health, disease: recent work on medieval women's medicine', *Studies in Medieval and Renaissance History*, third series, 2 (2005), 1-46.

order of being born'.[27] Similar language can be found in the account of Hermengard, who claimed that her premature baby girl had been 'born against the laws of nature'.[28] This clearly elucidates a conviction that there was a natural, expected method of giving birth, deviations from which could be identified by female attendants or by the expectant mothers themselves.

Complementing this notion of a natural progression of events, the *Miracula* reveal the idea that there was a natural state of health. Illness and disease were considered to be a deviation from this natural physical condition. The lengthier account of St Edmund's miracles describes the languor experienced by a woman named Cristiana: 'her entire body was exhausted by the deterioration, forsaken by the powers of nature. Thus, with the natural powers overcome, she began gradually to languish'.[29] This idea of a deviation or loss of an expected physical state can also be found in the narratives of childbirth mentioned above. The women assisting Maria, while attempting to reposition the infant inside her womb, saw the body of the child 'in a heap of degenerating nature'.[30] The concept of a natural condition was evoked once again in the account of Hermengard's premature delivery. To the astonishment of both mother and midwife, Hermengard had produced a tiny infant, the size only of the midwife's hand, 'a shapeless thing', 'not of human appearance', 'an imperfection of nature'.[31]

Nature was presented in the miracle collections as a presumed typical standard to which an event or object customarily conformed. Yet, these standards were not considered to be rigid and unbreakable. Nature aimed for a benchmark, but had the potential to miss this mark, producing imperfections like the premature infants described by St Edmund's hagiographer. The physical world was not considered to be autonomous from the

[27] Cont[ra] modum parientium & ordinem nascentium nasci incipientem. Auxerre 123G, fol. 137vb.
[28] Contra jura nature natio. Auxerre 123G, fol. 132ra.
[29] Totum corpus ip[s]ius macie confectum, nature virib[us] destituitur. Ita q[uo]d naturalibus succumbentib[us] virib[us] cepit sensim languescere. Auxerre 123G, fol. 135va.
[30] In congeriem nature degenera[n]tis esse. Auxerre 123G, fol. 137vb.
[31] Res informis, nec erat species hominis, inp[er]fectio nature. Auxerre 123G, fol. 132ra.

intervention of God. Scriptural precedent and patristic writings supplied medieval authors with an interpretation of the world in which the natural order of events was prone to intrusions by portents, magic, marvels and miracles.[32] Indeed, St Edmund's miraculous intrusions were frequently portrayed as a rectification of the imperfections of nature, restoring the afflicted individual to a natural condition. Hermengard's tiny infant was 'granted by grace what indeed she was denied by nature' and revived from death long enough to be Baptised.[33] A similar example can be found in the account of the cure of an eight-year-old boy, described as 'a defect of nature'.[34] Once at the threshold of Pontigny Abbey, 'grace began to work in the boy that which could not be completed by nature'.[35] A miracle served to amend the failure of nature to achieve its typical standard and to restore the stricken individual to a natural state of health.[36] Although the cause of a miracle ultimately lay beyond the natural world, in God and His saints, a miracle operated to restore afflicted postulants to a natural state of health.

It is worth considering where our authors acquired their ideas about the functioning of the natural world and the role of the miraculous within this natural order. The beliefs about the natural order of events presented in St Edmund's *Miracula* were developed from observations made during everyday life. Hagiographers drew on their audience's personal experiences of consistent and regular patterns inherent in the natural world to validate their claims for a miracle. When recounting stories of the resurrection of dead individuals, the author of St Edmund's longer *Miracula* provided considerable details about the condition of the deceased and any tests employed to determine whether he or she was actually dead.

---

[32] Darren Oldridge, *Strange Histories: The Trial of the Pig, the Walking Dead and other Matters of Fact from the Medieval and Renaissance Worlds* (Abingdon, 2005), 8-9. For more on marvels and prodigies see Chris Given-Wilson, *Chronicles: The Writing of History in Medieval England* (London, 2004), 21-56.

[33] Conceditur a gr[ati]a q[uo] quidem erat denegatu[m] a natura. Auxerre 123G, fol. 132ra.

[34] Defec[tu]m nat[ur]e. Auxerre 123G, fol. 149vb.

[35] Cepit in puero gr[ati]a operari q[uo]d a natura no[n] poterat [con]summari. Auxerre 123G, fol. 149vb.

[36] Also see Walker Bynum, 'Miracles and marvels', 809.

In one such account, a widow named Agnes returned to her home only to discover that her young son had died in her absence. The author described the signs of death in great detail: the boy's eyes were open, his limbs rigid and his body cold. It was also reported that Agnes had placed her hand over her son's mouth for some time and observed no breath.[37] A similar level of detail can be found in the account of a boy named Odinus, who had drowned after having fallen into a deep waterlogged hole. Following his removal from the water, the accident-prone youngster was described as having a bluish complexion and a swollen, rigid and cold body. Furthermore, the observers noted that, 'no voice was in him, and no sensation, and no breath of life could be perceived in him'.[38] The hagiographer implicitly relied upon his audience's familiarity with certain recognised signs of death to convince them that the recipients of these miracles had actually been dead and consequently miraculously resurrected by St Edmund.[39]

The physical signs of death would have been familiar to medieval men and women through their activities preparing the bodies of the dead for burial. St Edmund's hagiographer provides evidence for this when reporting the reaction of Dana's neighbours to the death of her son. The women present in the house after little John's death were engaged in sewing his body into a cloth shroud when the boy miraculously revived.[40] Interestingly, in a deposition on this same miracle, recorded in St Edmund's canonization proceedings, John's brother Guy, also close at hand, was able to describe his brother's appearance and the behaviour of those present in the moments after death.[41] A result of this familiarity

---

[37] Auxerre 123G, fols 132ra-rb.

[38] Non erat in eo vox neq[ue] sensus, neq[ue] flatus vitalis in eo poterat perpendi. Auxerre 123G, fol. 150vb. For more on witnesses describing the physical indicators of death see Goodich, *Miracles and Wonders*, 94-99.

[39] On the difficulties experienced when attempting to establish death see Ronald Finucane, *Miracles and Pilgrims: Popular Beliefs in Medieval England* (London, 1977), 73-74.

[40] Auxerre 123G, fol. 124va.

[41] Jean-Luc Benoit, *Pontigny, Saint Edme, les moines et leurs voisins: L'abbaye cistercienne pendant la première moitié du XIIIe siècle*, volume 2 (Paris, 1997), 383-84. I am much obliged to Dr Benoit for allowing me access to his

with the bodies of the recently deceased implies that a variety of people, from the immediate family and beyond, would have been able to recognise the physical indicators of death from personal experience.[42]

The clerical authors of St Edmund's miracle collections may also have had access to a considerable literature describing the signs of death, found in both Latin and vernacular texts from the twelfth century onwards. Medical works, like Maurus of Salerno's commentary on the *Prognostics* of Hippocrates, provided information on the prognostic signs of death.[43] Vernacular manuscripts listing the signs of impending death, for either medical or spiritual purposes (to allow adequate time for repentance), appeared in Middle English from the twelfth century. Indeed, a thirteenth-century prose poem lists signs similar to those in St Edmund's accounts, including stiff feet, a cold nose and black lips, as just some of the indicators that death was approaching.[44]

The conception of a natural world containing characteristic and predictable patterns based on knowledge derived from commonplace experiences can be found in other thirteenth-century writings. Historians focusing on the themes of doubt and scepticism in medieval societies have identified the presence of this type of rationalistic explanation of everyday phenomena amongst the lower social strata. In his examination of inquisition depositions from Toulouse, generated between 1270 and 1273, Walter Wakefield identified materialist and pragmatic interpretations of natural occurrences, such as the attribution of plant growth to the

 transcript of one of the surviving fragments of the records of St Edmund's canonization enquiry, Sens: Cathédrale Saint-Étienne, Trésor Manuscript H22, and for his kind assistance at the Public Library in Auxerre.

[42] Also see Christopher Daniell, *Death and Burial in Medieval England, 1066 - 1550* (New York, 1997), 30-31 and 37.

[43] Morris H. Saffron, *Maurus of Salerno: Twelfth-Century 'Optimus physicus' with his Commentary on the Prognostics of Hippocrates* (Philadelphia, 1972), 83.

[44] Rossell H. Robbins, 'Signs of death in middle English', *Medieval Studies*, 32 (1970), 291. Rosemary Horrox, 'Purgatory, prayer and plague 1150-1380', in *Death in England*, edited by Peter C. Jupp and Clare Gittings (Manchester, 1999), 98-99. For the later middle ages see Eamon Duffy, *The Stripping of the Altars: Traditional Religion in England 1400-1580* (Yale, 1992), 310-13.

qualities of seed and soil rather than to God's direct intervention.[45] Similarly, Susan Reynolds argued that it was quite possible that individuals made common-sense distinctions between events which seemed to follow a natural course and those that did not.[46]

The nature of the source material available to historians, whether based on the analysis of sermon material, heresy trials or hagiography, makes it difficult to identify and investigate a 'popular' concept of nature.[47] The documentation we must rely on was produced by the clerical elite with a view to promoting their own agenda, rather than recording 'popular' ideas. Despite this, ideas about nature, which were based on knowledge derived from a direct experience of the natural order, are likely to have informed both the audience and the author of hagiographical works. After all, the provision of specific details describing a corpse would not have served as a believable indicator of death unless both the author and his audience trusted that these signs were reliable proofs of death.

Analysis of the language and ideas contained in St Edmund's miracle collections reveals another potential influence on the authors' conceptions of the natural and the miraculous. St Edmund's *Miracula* were influenced by an intellectual approach to the natural world formulated by twelfth-century scholars. Twelfth-century authors exhibited a growing interest in the natural world. Monastic writers and poets, like Alain of Lille and Bernard Sylvester, utilised allegories and personifications of nature in their

---

[45] Walter L. Wakefield, 'Some unorthodox popular ideas of the thirteenth century', *Medievalia et Humanistica*, 4 (1973), 29-33.

[46] Susan Reynolds, 'Social mentalities and the cases of medieval scepticism', *Transactions of the Royal Historical Society*, sixth series, 1 (1991), 30. Also see: Alexander Murray, 'Piety and impiety in thirteenth-century Italy', in *Popular Belief and Practice*, edited by Geoffrey J. Cuming and Derek Baker, Studies in Church History, 8 (Cambridge, 1972), 83-106; Carl Watkins, 'Providence, experience and doubt in the middle ages', in *Fictions of Knowledge: Fact, Evidence, Doubt*, edited by Yota Batsaki, Subha Mukherji and Jan-Melissa Schramm (Houndmills, Basingstoke, 2012), 40-60.

[47] For more on the problematised dichotomy between 'popular' and 'elite' beliefs see: Peter Brown, *The Cult of Saints: Its Rise and Function in Latin Christianity* (London, 1981), 17-20; Alexander Murry, *Reason and Society in the Middle Ages* (Oxford, 1978), 14-17; Watkins, *History and the Supernatural*, 5-12.

writings.⁴⁸ Accompanying this was a more literal interest in the natural world, identified in the works of scholars interested in medicine, astrology and mathematics.⁴⁹ Exposure to the writings of twelfth-century authors contained in the Pontigny Abbey Library and, for Albert of Armagh, experience of scholastic education at the University of Paris equipped our authors with a conception of a semi-autonomous natural order and provided the terminology through which they could discuss the workings of the natural world.

Archbishop Albert had studied at the University of Paris where natural philosophical writings featured in the curriculum of the faculty of arts.⁵⁰ Latin translations of Greek and Arabic works based on Aristotle's natural philosophy served as the curriculum for the arts faculties of thirteenth-century universities, including Paris.⁵¹ The arts degree was a prerequisite for matriculation to the higher degrees of medicine, law and theology, ensuring that theologians, canonists and physicians gained exposure to at least some of these ideas about the natural world.⁵² Albert of Armagh's direct exposure to Aristotle's writings may have been limited as a result of the 1210 edict prohibiting both public and private lecturing on Aristotle's natural philosophical works.⁵³ Nevertheless, an increased awareness

---

⁴⁸ French and Cunningham, *Before Science*, 75. Winthrop Wetherbee, *Platonism and Poetry in the Twelfth Century: The Literary Influence of the School of Chartres* (Princeton, 1972).

⁴⁹ French and Cunningham, *Before Science*, 73. Alistair C. Crombie, *Robert Grosseteste and the Origins of Experimental Science* (Oxford, 1953), 16-24.

⁵⁰ Friedrich W. Bautz, 'Albert II (Suerbeer)', in *Biographisch-Bibliographisches Kirchenlexikon*, volume 1 (Hamm, Westfalia, 1975), col. 84.

⁵¹ Norman Kretzmann. 'Aristotle in the middle ages', in *The Cambridge History of Later Medieval Philosophy: From the Rediscovery of Aristotle to the Disintegration of Scholasticism, 1100-1600*, edited by Norman Kretzmann, Anthony Kenny and Jan Pinborg (Cambridge, 1982), 48, 52.

⁵² Edward Grant, *God and Reason in the Middle Ages* (Cambridge, 2001), 101.

⁵³ Bernard G. Dod, '*Aristotles Latinus*', in *The Cambridge History of Later Medieval Philosophy: From the Rediscovery of Aristotle to the Disintegration of Scholasticism, 1100-1600*, edited by Norman Kretzmann, Anthony Kenny and Jan Pinborg (Cambridge, 1982), 48. The effectiveness of the prohibition has been questioned by David Lindberg; see David C. Lindberg, *The Beginnings of Western Science: The European Scientific Tradition in Philosophical, Religious and Institutional Context 600 BC to AD 1450* (Chicago and London, 1992), 217.

of the regularity of the natural order was already present in the writings of twelfth-century scholars, writings available at the universities and at Pontigny Abbey itself.

Analysis of the Latin terminology used by the authors of St Edmund's miracle narratives to describe the natural world reveals a conception of nature inherited from writings composed in the twelfth-century monasteries and schools. Our hagiographers' characterisation of miracles as '*contra naturam*' and description of problematic births as either '*contra modum et ordinem nature*' or '*contra iura nature*' can also be found in writings available in the library at Pontigny.[54] The library catalogues which record works kept at the abbey reveal the existence of a twelfth-century manuscript of Peter Lombard's *Sentences*, along with John of Salisbury's *Policraticus* and Adelard of Bath's *Questiones naturales*.[55] These works provided access to twelfth-century scholarly ideas about nature, which articulated a belief that God had provided the world with a rationalistic structure with the capacity to operate by its own laws.[56]

The writings of these twelfth-century scholars must be situated within the broader development of ideas about the natural world, since their articulation of a belief in a predictable natural order represented a reworking of pre-existing ideas about the natural world. The predominant influence on attitudes to nature before the twelfth century was Plato's *Timaeus*, the first book of which was available in western Christian Europe through Calcidius's fourth-century translation, accompanied by his commentary on the text.[57] This tradition had been received by patristic authorities, including St Augustine and St Ambrose, who handed down to later generations the idea of nature as a complex series of causes able to

---

[54] Auxerre 123G, fols 105rb, 126ra, 132ra, 137vb and 149va.
[55] Peyrafort-Huin, *La Bibliothèque*, 81.
[56] Grant, *God and Reason*, 72.
[57] Charles Burnett, 'Scientific speculations', in *A History of Twelfth-Century Western Philosophy*, edited by Peter Dronke (Cambridge, 1988), 168. Benedict M. Ashley OP, 'St Albert and the nature of natural science', in *Albertus Magnus and the Sciences: Commemorative Essays*, edited by James A. Weisheipl (Toronto, 1980), 74.

function without the direct interference of God.[58] Augustine situated the miraculous within this concept of nature, arguing that a miracle was often the result of the acceleration of properties inherent in an object, of 'seminal causes' or seeds built into the material world by its Creator and later activated.[59] Miracles were not contrary to nature as all acts of the creator were considered natural and all had their origin in the greatest miracle, that of creation itself. St Augustine made this clear in his influential fifth-century work, *The City of God against the Pagans*: 'men say that all portents are contrary to nature. They are not so, however; for how is that contrary to nature which happens by the will of God, since the will of so great a Creator is certainly the nature of every created thing?'[60] St Augustine went on to explain that although certain events were not contrary to nature, they could appear to be contrary to what was *known* of nature.[61]

The twelfth-century works of Peter Lombard, John of Salisbury and Adelard of Bath demonstrate a shift in these ideas, with a much greater emphasis being placed on the secondary causes of events and the influence of processes within the natural world.[62] The idea that nature provided predictable patterns perceived through experience can be clearly seen in John of Salisbury's *Policraticus*.[63] Here, John defined nature as 'the customary course of events and the hidden causes of phenomena for which a reasonable explanation can be given'.[64] When discussing omens, John of

---

[58] Tullio Gregory, 'The platonic inheritance', in *A History of Twelfth-Century Western Philosophy*, edited by Peter Dronke (Cambridge, 1988), 63.

[59] Goodich, *Miracles and Wonders*, 14.

[60] Augustine, *The City of God against the Pagans*, edited and translated by Robert W. Dyson (Cambridge, 1998), 1061.

[61] Goodich, *Miracles and Wonders*, 13-14. Augustine, *City of God*, 1061.

[62] Ward, *Miracles and the Medieval Mind*, 6.

[63] For an assessment of the influence of Aristotle on John of Salisbury's *Metalogicon*, see Charles Burnett, 'John of Salisbury and Aristotle', *Didascalia*, 1 (1996), 19-32.

[64] Dum tamen naturam hic, ut in locis quam pluribus dicamus solitum cursum rerum, aut causas occultas euentuum, quarum ratio reddi potest. *Ioannis Saresberiensis episcopi Carnotensis Policratici*, volume 1, edited by Clement C. I. Webb (Oxford, 1909), 85. Joseph B. Pike, *Frivolities of the Courtiers and Footprints of Philosophers: Being a Translation of the First, Second and Third Books of the Policraticus of John of Salisbury* (London, 1938), 73.

Salisbury declared that, if nature was viewed as the common course of things, some occurrences could be considered *contra naturam*. Yet, he qualified this statement by adding that if nature was seen as the will of God, then nothing could be *contra naturam*.[65] This common course of events could be observed by physicians, who 'learn to recognise the imminence of health, disease or the state they term neutral or even death itself by preceding symptoms ... the judgement they pronounce as the result of their knowledge of symptoms, though attained with difficulty, often proves exceptionally sound'.[66] For John of Salisbury observing the world could lead to knowledge of its inherent order. That said, John of Salisbury was also wary of over-extending these naturalising interpretations of the world, denouncing certain physicians who, by 'placing undue emphasis upon nature, in general encroach upon the rights of the author of nature by their opposition to faith'.[67] Our author was acutely aware of the need to maintain the conceptual capacity for divine intervention in the world. The *Policraticus*, it is worth noting, does not contain a thoroughly formulated conception of nature, though it does show the interaction, not always harmonious, of Platonic and Augustinian ideas about nature with a twelfth-century desire to elucidate the predictable natural order within the world.

The desires of twelfth-century scholars to provide naturalistic explanations for occurrences led to attempts to attribute causes to God only when these expositions failed. This approach was

---

[65] Si uero Platonem sequimur qui asserit naturam esse Dei uoluntatem, profecto nichil istorum euenit contra naturam. Webb, *Ioannis Saresberiensis*, 85. For a detailed analysis of the varied meanings of the phrase *contra naturam* in its political and legal context see Jacques Chiffoleau, '*Contra naturam*: pour une approche caustique et procédurale de la nature médiévale', *Micrologus*, 4 (1996), 265-312.

[66] Ars phisicorum regulis suis satis probabiliter comprehendit futuram etiam sanitatem egritudinem aut statum quem dicunt neutralitatem, fatalitatem quoque ipsam ex praecedentibus signis agnoscunt, et interdum si causas nouerint, efficacissime curant ... iudicium uero, quod ex signorum cognitione proferunt, etsi difficile, saepe verissimum est. Webb, *Ioannis Saresberiensis*, 69. Pike, *Policraticus*, 58-59.

[67] Dum naturae nimium auctoritatis attribuunt, in auctorem naturea aduersando fidei plerumque impingunt. Webb, *Ioannis Saresberiensis*, 167. Pike, *Policraticus*, 149.

articulated in the work of Adelard of Bath, who sought to explain phenomena without immediate recourse to God.[68] In his *Questiones naturales*, when discussing the composition of celestial bodies, Adelard declared that 'in every discussion it is most important to consider the nature of that which is discussed. For nothing reveals the consequent effects of anything better than the composition of that thing's own essence (leaving aside the inexplicable contribution of the efficient cause)', that is, leaving aside God.[69] These naturalising methods were even deemed appropriate as a technique for scriptural analysis. In the *Policraticus*, John of Salisbury assessed biblical signs in terms of whether they violated nature's laws. He declared that the eclipse of the sun at the crucifixion could not have been a natural one since it occurred at a time when an eclipse was not to be expected.[70]

Restricting the definition of nature to the common course of events and placing greater emphasis on secondary causes meant that it was possible that some occurrences could genuinely take place against nature, in contrast with St Augustine's earlier postulations. Peter Lombard followed the Augustinian idea of seminal causes, that some causes were naturally occurring, yet he augmented this argument by proposing that some causes lay beyond nature (*preter naturam*) and could be attributed to God alone.[71] Lombard's *Sentences* received a wide distribution in the twelfth and thirteenth centuries and was later adopted as a textbook at the University of Paris by Alexander of Hales.[72] It is worth noting that language

---

[68] Lindberg, *The Beginnings of Western Science*, 200. Bert Hansen, *Nicole Oresme and the Marvels of Nature: A Study of his 'De causis mirabilium' with Critical Edition, Translation and Commentary* (Toronto, 1985), 55.

[69] Adelard of Bath, *Conversations with his Nephew: 'On the Same and the Different', 'Questions on Natural Science', and 'On Birds'*, edited by Charles Burnett (Cambridge, 1998), 221.

[70] Webb, *Ioannis Saresberiensis*, 84. Pike, *Policraticus*, 72. Also see Walker Bynum, 'Miracles and marvels', 808.

[71] Bartlett, *Natural and the Supernatural*, 6.

[72] Grant, *God and Reason*, 210. Alexander of Hales, whose teachings and work at Oxford and Paris were at the cutting edge of thirteenth-century theological scholarship, was called on by the Pope to participate in St Edmund's canonization process. Other theologians involved in St Edmund's canonization included Cardinal John of Toledo, a Master in theology and student of medicine and Robert Grosseteste, Bishop of Lincoln, who had

referring to seminal causes and deeds that were *preter naturam* does not appear in either of St Edmund's miracle collections. From the multitude of approaches and ideas about nature available in the second quarter of the thirteenth century, St Edmund's hagiographers adopted the phrase, *contra naturam*, which indicated simply that an event occurred against the course of nature, without qualifying this phenomenon further.

Furthermore, the authors of St Edmund's miracle collections were provided with the language and terminology through which to discuss the natural world by earlier hagiographical texts. Nestled amongst the numerous patristic and biblical texts kept at Pontigny Abbey was a copy of Benedict of Peterborough's *Passion of St Thomas*.[73] On several occasions this late twelfth-century work referred to imperfections of nature, employing the same language as St Edmund's anonymous hagiographer. Benedict of Peterborough described a young boy named Henry as 'an imperfection of nature', while a woman named Agnes displayed 'a form of degenerating nature'.[74] As we have seen, similar phrases echo throughout St Edmund's lengthier miracle collection. A prematurely born infant was 'disfigured by a strange imperfection of nature', while another hapless neonate was described as 'an imperfection of nature'.[75] Correspondingly, the horribly swollen body of a woman from Villa Nova, according to the hagiographer, 'displayed a form of degenerating nature'.[76] The terminology used to express the idea

lectured at Oxford in theology and whose writings showed the influence of Aristotelian and Neoplatonic ideas. Lawrence, *The Life of St Edmund*, 97. Also see Wilfried Hartmann and Kenneth Pennington, *The History of Medieval Canon Law in the Classical Period, 1140-1234: From Gratian to the Decretals of Pope Gregory IX* (Washington DC, 2008), 231. Alistair C. Crombie, *Science, Art and Nature in Medieval and Modern Thought* (London, 1996), 39-44. For more on the involvement of theologians in canonization proceedings see Goodich, *Miracles and Wonders*, 26.

[73] Peyrafort-Huin, *La Bibliothèque*, 90.

[74] Imperfectio nature. Nature degenerantis formam preferebat. Benedict of Peterborough, *'Passio Sancti Thomae Cantuariensis'*, in *Materials for the History of Thomas Becket, Archbishop of Canterbury*, edited by James C. Robertson, volume 2, Rolls Series (London, 1875-85), 88-89, 68.

[75] Mira inp[er]fect[i]one nature deturpatum. Auxerre 123G, fol. 149rb. Erat inp[er]fectio nature. Auxerre 123G, fol. 131vb.

[76] Nature degenerantis formam preferebat. Auxerre 123G, fol. 126va. Also see Auxerre 123G, fols 137vb and 130va.

that nature was prone to imperfections had been present in hagiographical writings dating from the late twelfth century, providing a model which St Edmund's hagiographer could choose to replicate.

The terminology used to discuss the natural and the non-natural in St Edmund's miracle accounts also corresponded to that used in chronicles, medical and natural philosophical writings. St Edmund's collection describes the method of childbirth experienced by Oudeburgis as '*innaturaliter*', because the mother emitted no cry during her labour. This term was used a second time to describe the newborn infant's 'little body', which was 'made unnaturally [*innaturaliter*] round'.[77] This expression can also be found in Walter Map's late twelfth-century work, *De nugis curialium* and in Gerald of Wales's *Topographia Hibernica*.[78] In a similar manner, the appearance of the adjectival form of this word, '*innaturalis*', entered into the vocabulary of thirteenth-century chroniclers like Matthew Paris and also appeared in medical writings compiled by both Bartholomaeus Anglicus and Gilbertus Anglicus.[79] Authors writing in the thirteenth century were able to draw on a wide and varied vocabulary about the natural world to describe the events and behaviours reported by healed pilgrims.

To summarise the argument so far, descriptions relating to the natural world appear throughout the accounts of St Edmund's miracles. These presented nature as an habitual sequence of events or an expected physical condition. A closer examination of the material contained in these miracle narratives indicates that ideas about the natural world were developed both from observations made during daily life and the influence of twelfth-century scholastic discourses about nature. Changes in perceptions of the natural world, which occurred during the twelfth century, filtered into the writings of thirteenth-century hagiographers, shaping their

---

[77] Corpusculum innaturaliter conglobatum. Auxerre 123G, fol. 130vb.

[78] Ronald E. Latham, *Dictionary of Medieval Latin* (London, 1975), 1387. Ronald E. Latham, *Revised Medieval Latin Wordlist from British and Irish Sources* (Oxford, 2004), 251.

[79] Bartholomaeus Anglicus, *De proprietatibus rerum* and Gilbertus Anglicus, *Compendium medicinae*. Latham, *Dictionary of Medieval Latin*, 1387. Matthew Paris, *Chronica majora*, edited by Henry Richards Luard, volume 3, Rolls Series (London, 1876), 519.

conception of the natural order and relocating the realm of the miraculous beyond this order. With these thoughts in mind the following subsection will consider how these ideas influenced the presentation of St Edmund's miracles. In particular, how the conceptual distinction between a natural occurrence and a miraculous event generated the need to eliminate possible natural causes in order to authenticate a miracle.

Against the Order of Nature: Authenticating St Edmund's Miracles

As we have seen, the restriction of the concept of nature to the typical operations of the natural world firmly positioned a miracle outside this natural order. Accordingly, it was imperative that St Edmund's hagiographers demonstrate that the specific events described did not have a natural basis. To achieve this, the writers emphasised that the recipient of a healing miracle did not have recourse to physical care, or, if they did, that these remedies were unsuccessful. They also relied on the diagnostic knowledge of physicians to verify that a condition could not be healed by earthly means. Furthermore, the appearance of medical discourses and humoral terminology within these works reveals an underlying acceptance of academic medicine as an explanatory framework for disease.

The author of St Edmund's lengthier *Miracula* dismissed the potential contribution of natural, earthly treatments for the recovery of a young boy. The boy's father had arranged for a surgeon to operate on the child. However, on discovering this, the youngster's grandmother reproached the surgeon and invoked St Edmund instead. The author assured his audience that 'we learn from visible signs and reliable evidence, [that] the boy was cured without human aid'.[80] Albert of Armagh adopted a similar argument when recounting the restoration of a mute Englishman named Walter. The Archbishop stressed the duration of Walter's illness, which had afflicted him continuously from birth for thirty-three years 'so that all hope of recovering speech by the benefit of

---

[80] Evidentib[us] signis et certis indiciis [con]perim[us] puerum sive humano subsidio sanari. Auxerre 123G, fol. 141va.

nature or art ... had been entirely removed'.[81] Both authors considered it necessary to demonstrate that a physical healing played no part in the recovery of St Edmund's postulants.

Where medicinal remedies had been applied, St Edmund's hagiographers asserted that these treatments had failed to heal their patients, again eliminating the possibility of a cure by natural means. This is most notable in a narrative reporting the cure of William, a young man from Paris. The recommendations of William's physicians to 'bathe his entire body in the salty waves of the sea' failed leaving him thoroughly disheartened.[82] Similarly reported were the unsuccessful efforts of a monk named Alanus, who had applied 'many medicaments' along with a multitude of remedies including herbal medicines in an effort to cure his deafness.[83] This emphasis on the failure of physical treatments served to eradicate the possibility that medicines had contributed to the removal of the condition, thereby establishing that the cure was of supernatural, rather than natural, origin.

A common trope in hagiographical works is the assertion that the treatments offered by physicians failed to cure their patients. This has habitually been viewed by historians as a critique of ineffective medical practitioners and as evidence for a conflict between the remedies offered by earthly healers and their heavenly counterparts.[84] While criticism of physicians and their remedies continues to feature in St Edmund's miracles, these thirteenth-century texts display a more detailed integration of medical discourses into writings about the miraculous. St Edmund's hagiographers' dismissal of the effectiveness of medical treatment can be viewed as an attempt to eliminate natural processes as the potential cause for an event, in order to confirm the miraculous

---

[81] Ita quod omnis spes recuperande loquele nature vel artis beneficio ... omnino sublata fuerat: Auxerre 123G, fols 109vb-110ra.

[82] Salsis fluctib[us] maris totu[m] corpus ablueret. Auxerre 123G, fol. 143ra.

[83] Plurima medicamina, medicinas plurimas herbarum. Auxerre 123G, fol. 150rb.

[84] Valerie Flint, 'The early medieval *medicus*, the saint and the enchanter', *Social History of Medicine*, 2 (1989), 136. Patricia Skinner, 'A cure for a sinner: sickness and healthcare in medieval southern Italy', in *The Community, the Family and the Saint: Patterns of Power in Early Medieval Europe*, edited by Joyce Hill and Mary Swan (Turnhout, 1998), 308.

origin of the cure. Rather than denigrating the utility of medical knowledge and physicians, the perceived need to reject the contribution of medicine perhaps reflects a belief that these remedies could in certain circumstances result in successful cures.

Moreover, our authors exploited the diagnostic expertise of physicians to validate the healing miracles which they described. This is particularly prominent in Albert of Armagh's *Miracula* which records that at least three of those who claimed to have experienced a miracle were called to testify before the Apostolic See and examined by physicians.[85] A woman named Adelina was summoned before the papal court to confirm her recovery from a contracted leg and an enormous hump on her back, conditions which Albert referred to as incurable. Once there she was 'strictly examined by the cardinals, by the Lord Pope himself and by his physicians', who touched the place where the hump had been and established that her health had not been restored by any natural means.[86] This was not unique to St Edmund's process. The early thirteenth-century *Book of St Gilbert* reports that several of St Gilbert's miracle recipients were summoned to the curia to give evidence before the pope.[87]

Reliance on the conclusions of physicians can also be found in St Edmund's anonymous *Miracula*. The physicians treating a certain Master Simon diagnosed the itching ulcers and pustules on his left hand as symptoms of the chronic illness St Antony's fire and advised that the hand be amputated to prevent the condition from

---

[85] Auxerre 123G, fols 106va-107ra. Also see fols 109vb-110rb and 111rb-112ra.

[86] A cardinalibus quam ab ipso domino papa & ejus medicis strictissime examinata. Auxerre 123G, fols 106vb-107ra. Agostino Paravicini-Bagliani has identified the attendance of more than seventy physicians serving popes and cardinals throughout the thirteenth century. Agostino Paravicini-Bagliani, *The Pope's Body*, translated by David S. Peterson (Chicago and London, 2000), 191-92. Also see James J. Walsh, *The Popes and Science* (New York, 1915), 205.

[87] Foreville and Keir, *The Book of St Gilbert*, 173. For more on the involvement of physicians in canonization processes see Joseph Ziegler, 'Practitioners and saints: medical men in canonization processes in the thirteenth to fifteenth centuries', *Social History of Medicine*, 12 (1999), 191-225.

spreading.⁸⁸ Luckily for Master Simon, such a drastic procedure was unnecessary as St Edmund intervened and healed the stricken limb, leaving only a blackish scar as evidence of the man's former affliction. A further example can be found in the narrative of Matheus, a nobleman cured by St Edmund from a quartan fever. Matheus had similarly 'consulted diligent physicians' who 'despairing, having given up hope, abandoned him, declaring him not able to be cured by a human hand'.⁸⁹ Confidence in the ability of physicians to judge the limits of medical healing and thus the boundaries of the natural world was displayed both by those involved in papal canonization enquiries and by the authors of hagiographical works.

In addition to this dependency on the prognostic and diagnostic abilities of physicians, medical learning featured in St Edmund's collections as an explanatory framework for disease. Our anonymous hagiographer displayed an understanding of humoral terminology and medical diagnostic knowledge through his description of the physical conditions afflicting St Edmund's ailing supplicants. The aforementioned knight Matheus was described as suffering 'from an increasing melancholy of the concoction of the blood'.⁹⁰ Melancholia, or black bile, was one of the four bodily fluids which was believed to constitute an individual's humoral complexion.⁹¹ This causal assessment was consistent with academic medical theory. The Muslim physician Ibn al-Jazzār, in his treatise on fevers, correspondingly ascribed the origin of a quartan fever to the putrefaction of black bile.⁹² This particular treatise, with its associated commentaries, was consulted widely during the

⁸⁸ Morbo cronico laborabat videlicet igne sancti antonii sive infernali. Auxerre 123G, fol. 146ra.

⁸⁹ Medicos industrios consuluit qui omnes desperantes desp[er]atum dimiserunt asserentes illu[m] non posse curari humana manu. Auxerre 123G, fol. 151rb.

⁹⁰ In crescente melancholia decocti sanguinis. Auxerre 123G, fols 151rb-va. For an explanation of the concoction of the blood within the organs see Nancy Siraisi, *Medieval and Early Renaissance Medicine: An Introduction to Knowledge and Practice* (Chicago, 1990), 106.

⁹¹ Siraisi, *Medieval and Early Renaissance Medicine*, 101-06. For further examples of humoral terminology see Auxerre 123G, fols 124ra, 124rb, 130va and 140ra.

⁹² Ibn al-Jazzār, *On Fevers*, translated by Gerrit Bos (London, 2000), 127.

thirteenth century due to its incorporation into the *Articella* – a compendium of medical texts which constituted the core of the medical curriculum.[93]

The explanatory authority of scholastic medicine and its practitioners was reinforced by the integration of natural philosophical ideas into the medieval medical corpus from the late eleventh century onwards.[94] The very ideas that operated to alter the twelfth- and thirteenth-century conception of the natural world were present in newly translated medical works. Medicine was one of the first branches of knowledge to benefit from the introduction of Islamic knowledge into the western world during the eleventh and twelfth centuries. Arabic works, like those by Avicenna and Averroes, both of whom were professionally engaged as physicians and philosophers, expanded the theoretical basis of western medicine, providing access to writings strongly influenced by Aristotelian doctrines.[95] As a result of their acquaintance with natural philosophy, physicians were uniquely placed to assess the boundaries of the natural world and the validity of miraculous cures.

The presence of humoral theory and citation of the opinions of physicians in St Edmund's *Miracula* perhaps reflects a heightened confidence in the authority of medical knowledge as an explanatory

---

[93] Siraisi, *Medieval and Early Renaissance Medicine*, 58. Alan B. Cobban, *The Medieval Universities: their Development and Organization* (London, 1975), 37-47. Paul O. Kristeller, 'Bartholomaeus, Musandinus, and Maurus of Salerno and other early commentators on the *Articella*, with a tentative list of manuscripts', *Italia Medioevale e Umanistica*, 19 (1976), 57-87. Charles Burnett, 'The institutional context of Arabic-Latin translations of the middle ages: a reassessment of the "School of Salerno"', in *Vocabulary of Teaching and Research between Middle Ages and Renaissance*, edited by Olga Weijers (Turnhout, 1995), 214-35.

[94] Modern scholars have noted the influence of Aristotelian ideas as early as the 1160s in the commentaries produced by the Salernitan masters Bartholomaeus, Maurus and Urso. French and Cunningham, *Before Science*, 89-90. For the influence of Aristotle on Maurus of Salerno see Saffron, *Maurus of Salerno*.

[95] Paul O. Kristeller, 'Philosophy and medicine in medieval and renaissance Italy', in *Organism, Medicine and Metaphysics*, edited by Stuart F. Spicker (Dordrech, 1978), 30-31.

model, which developed during the mid-thirteenth century.[96] It is no coincidence that the involvement of doctors as expert testators in canonization proceedings coexisted with their increased participation in civil law cases to judge the severity of injuries sustained during physical assault.[97] Experience of the involvement of physicians during St Edmund's canonization process may itself have reinforced the authority of scholastic medicine as method of establishing the limits of natural causation. At the root of this reliance on both medical theory and the prognostic capabilities of physicians to authenticate miracles was an assumption that the intended audience for the *Miracula* shared the authors' confidence in the ability of medicine to assess the limits of the natural world.

This examination of the miracle collections of St Edmund of Abingdon has demonstrated the ways in which twelfth-century modifications in the understanding of nature influenced the definition of a miracle among thirteenth-century hagiographers. God's interventions within the world became confined to those deeds which could not be explained by secondary causes and thus occurred against the perceived order inherent in the observable world. These ideas were disseminated to clerical audiences, including St Edmund's hagiographers, accentuating the need for them to eliminate potential natural causes for alleged miraculous cures. The authors achieved this in three ways: first, by reassuring their audience that no medicines had been applied, second, by asserting that, even if medicines had been applied, they had failed to have any effect, and finally by claiming that physicians believed that the condition was incurable.

St Edmund's miracle collections reflect the ways in which natural philosophical and medical concepts became integrated into the writings of scholars based outside the universities and monastic schools of western Europe. Authors responded to developing scholastic definitions of the natural and supernatural worlds

---

[96] Michael R. McVaugh, *Medicine before the Plague: Practitioners and their Patients in the Crown of Aragon, 1285-1345* (Cambridge, 1993), 190-91. For the status of English physicians in the later middle age see Carole Rawcliffe, 'The profits of practice: the wealth and status of medical men in later medieval England', *Social History of Medicine*, 1 (1998), 61-78.

[97] McVaugh, *Medicine Before the Plague*, 207-08.

acquired from earlier writings and practical experience. These conclusions highlight the need to examine the range of ideas informing the authors of hagiographical texts, including, as this study has shown, an author's intellectual background and the place of composition. Furthermore, the existence of partial records for St Edmund's canonization process raises further questions, beyond the scope of this present study, about the influence of the evidential requirements of the canonization process on the hagiographical texts composed before and after these enquiries. In assessing St Edmund's *Miracula*, I hope to have provided a glimpse into the conception of the miraculous articulated by those directly engaged in the promotion of miracles and to have provided evidence for the assimilation of natural philosophy and medical knowledge into thirteenth-century clerical texts.

'CHRIST MORE POWERFUL THAN GALEN'? THE RELATIONSHIP BETWEEN MEDICINE AND MIRACLES

Iona McCleery

In the mid-thirteenth-century Dominican *Lives of the Brethren*, it was reported that Gil de Santarém, Portuguese friar and former physician (d. 1265):

> encouraged the sick, although he himself was often sick, with his consoling advice, warning that they should not treat themselves with medicines, but with faith in Christ they should joyfully accept what was served them and it would benefit them greatly, because grace is stronger than nature, and Christ more powerful than Galen.[1]

Historians would once have taken these words at face value and understood Gil's words to mean a denigration of human medicine, represented by the famous ancient authority Galen, and the exaltation of divine healing, represented by Christ. Many medical historians would now argue for a more symbiotic relationship between medicine and religion, based on a nuanced analysis of a wider range of narrative and archival sources, including hagiography.[2] Careful analysis of Gil's own life and his highly

---

[1] *Vitae fratrum ordinis praedicatorum*, edited by Benedict Maria Reichert, *Monumenta ordinis fratrum praedicatorum historica*, volume 1 (Louvain, 1896), 155 (my translation).

[2] Joseph Ziegler, *Medicine and Religion c.1300: The Case of Arnau de Vilanova* (Oxford, 1998); *Religion and Medicine in the Middle Ages*, edited by Peter Biller and Joseph Ziegler (Woodbridge, 2001); John Henderson, *The Renaissance Hospital: Healing the Body and Healing the Soul* (New Haven and London, 2006); Angela Montford, *Health, Sickness, Medicine and the Friars in the Thirteenth and Fourteenth Centuries* (Aldershot, 2004); Peregrine Horden, *Hospitals and Healing from Antiquity to the Later Middle Ages* (Aldershot, 2008).

medicalized miracles, suggests that for him too, the relationship between Christ and Galen was really rather complex.³

Over the last thirty years medical historians have grown increasingly confident in their use of medieval miracle accounts and saints' lives as sources for medical practice, the experience of illness, and the medicalization of society. However, there is no systematic study of the relationship between medical and miraculous evidence for the middle ages, and it remains a neglected area of research particularly amongst late medievalists working on the history of medicine. There are cults from many parts of Europe that have yet to be studied much at all, let alone investigated for what they could reveal about the multi-faceted relationship between medicine and religion. This essay asks the following questions: what has the word 'medicine' meant to those studying healing cults at different times? What are the most useful methods for analysing miraculous healing? How can historians studying miracles in diverse parts of Europe (and the world) use methods developed for completely different cultural contexts? As case studies the essay introduces three little-known Portuguese healing cults: the aforementioned cult of Gil de Santarém, the cult of Our Lady of the Olive Tree from Guimarães in northern Portugal and the Holy Name of Jesus from Lisbon.

What is Medicine?

Before we begin, it is important to reflect on what constitutes 'medicalization' and indeed 'medicine' when studying healing miracles. 'Medicalization' refers to the widening use of medical vocabulary and the widespread involvement of medical practitioners in diagnosis and treatment. Even if they are said to have failed, medical practitioners and their diagnoses and therapies often played a prominent role in miracles. Furthermore, as Joseph Ziegler has shown, it was in the thirteenth century that physicians and surgeons began to take up the role they enjoy today as expert

---

[3] Iona McCleery, 'Saintly physician, diabolical doctor, medieval saint: exploring the reputation of Gil de Santarém in medieval and renaissance Portugal', *Portuguese Studies*, 21 (2005), 112-25.

witnesses in canonization processes.[4] 'Medicine' is more difficult to define. At a recent conference the present author delivered a paper on the healing miracles of Isabel of Aragon, queen of Portugal (d. 1336), relating how Isabel healed a leper of a head wound by applying an egg-white plaster. This example was put forward as evidence for Isabel's medical practice.[5] Afterwards, a woman in the audience denied that this was an example of medicine: instead it was 'just what women did'. Isabel's healing practice was deemed to be non-professional and therefore not medicine.

This experience led to some reflection over whether medieval men and women differed in their healing practices, both as medical practitioners and as saints. Monica Green has pioneered the study of gendered healthcare and there has been a great deal of work on gender and saints.[6] Yet the realisation came that many scholars interested in miracles are not actually very interested in healing *per se*; they tend to see the miracle as the unstable category that requires rationalising, not 'medicine'.[7] Ronald Finucane observed in a paper published in 1975 that 'the problem is not the definition of

[4] Joseph Ziegler, 'Practitioners and saints: medical men in canonization processes in the thirteenth to fifteenth centuries', *Social History of Medicine*, 12 (1999), 191-225.

[5] 'Vida e milagres de Dona Isabel, rainha de Portugal', edited by José Joaquim Nunes, *Boletim da segunda classe da Academia das Sciências de Lisboa*, 13 (1918-19), 1378-79.

[6] Monica Green, 'Gendering the history of women's healthcare', *Gender and History*, 20 (2008), 487-518; *Gender and Holiness: Men, Women and Saints in Late Medieval Europe*, edited by Samantha Riches and Sarah Salih (London, 2002); Sari Katajala-Peltomaa, *Gender, Miracles and Daily Life: The Evidence of Fourteenth-Century Canonization Processes* (Turnhout, 2009).

[7] It is actually quite unusual for hagiographical studies to analyse illness and healing in much detail. For example, Katajala-Peltomaa, *Gender, Miracles and Daily Life*, hardly mentions them, and nor does Steven Justice, 'Did the middle ages believe in their miracles?', *Representations*, 103 (2008), 1-29. Rachel Koopmans, *Wonderful to Relate: Miracle Stories and Miracle Collecting in High Medieval England* (Philadelphia, 2011), and Simon Yarrow, *Saints and their Communities: Miracle Stories in Twelfth Century England* (Oxford, 2006), are interested in healing, but it is not the focus of their studies. There is a chapter on healing in *The Cambridge Companion to Miracles*, edited by Graham H. Twelftree (Cambridge, 2011), but it focuses on miraculous belief in modern clinical practice. For a much fuller analysis of the meaning of miracles, including healing miracles, see now Robert Bartlett, *Why Can the Dead Do Such Great Things? Saints and Worshippers from the Martyrs to the Reformation* (Princeton, 2013), 349-64.

'miracle' ... it is a question of the definition of health and illness'.[8] Finucane did not problematise medicine; in much of his work he explained away miracle cures by resorting to modern theories of remission, vitamin deficiency and psycho-somatic illness.[9] However, his point still stands. We are not much closer to reaching a consensus on what health and illness were in the middle ages, how effective medieval people were at restoring the one and preventing the other from occurring, and indeed whether effectiveness is even an appropriate question to ask our sources. Yet from the perspective of hagiographical studies, medicine can sometimes be taken as a given, especially in contrast to the apparently 'irrational' miracles that are the focus of study.

When historians began to study miracle cults more carefully, it was the cults that acquired social functions and explanations, not medicine.[10] Yet medicine is an untidy 'umbrella' concept, not a neat category. In the UK today it includes GPs, nurses, hospitals, university teaching and research, blood banks, organ donation, medical charities, dentists, chemists and opticians, drug companies, public health policy, personal hygiene, sex education, diet and exercise, alternative therapies, environmental health, and health insurance. All these things have multiple functions and require a great deal of explanation. Since the 1980s there have been fundamental changes to our modern understanding of life, death, disease and cures. We are less confident in our ability to annihilate disease, less confident about whether our longer lives are healthier, while across the world people are still paying the health cost of colonialism. Globally there is a lack of consensus about the best system of entitlement to healthcare. All these things affect how we

---

[8] Ronald C. Finucane, 'The use and abuse of medieval miracles', *History*, 60 (1975), 6.

[9] Ronald C. Finucane, *Miracles and Pilgrims: Popular Beliefs in Medieval England* (New York, 1995); Ronald C. Finucane, *The Rescue of the Innocents: Endangered Children in Medieval Miracles* (New York, 2000).

[10] The pioneer of the functional approach to saints' cults was Peter Brown, *The Cult of the Saints: Its Rise and Function in Latin Christianity* (Chicago, 1981). See also the essays by Anne E. Bailey and Simon Yarrow in this volume.

study past lives and we should reflect on them more than we currently do. Medicine must not be taken for granted.[11]

Taking medicine for granted has tended to result in the preservation of attitudes present in the miracle narratives themselves, that is, that there was conflict or competition between medicine and religion. Gil de Santarém's reported comment about the power of Christ over that of Galen is a good example of such a medieval attitude. Other examples are the many cases in miracles where doctors failed to cure illnesses later healed by the saint, a topos that goes back to the Bible. There is no full-length study of medieval miracles that investigates these conflicts from a medical perspective. Perhaps surprisingly, though, there is now a study of modern miracles that does just that. In Jacalyn Duffin's analysis of over 1400 miracles from 374 beatification and canonization processes between 1588 and 1999, medicine is not taken for granted. In fact, for Duffin, miracles are an important source for how and why medical knowledge and practices were constructed, challenged, contested and adopted over the centuries, changing and spreading globally as time went on. Duffin, who is a practising haematologist as well as a noted historian of nineteenth-century clinical medicine, concludes that medicine and religion are heavily intertwined constructs or belief systems that equally demand and challenge the faith of their adherents and practitioners.[12] These demands compete with each other, therefore setting up an apparent opposition between the two belief systems which is imbedded in the system through teleological narratives produced 'in-house'. Gil de Santarém's reported speech makes sense within an intensely pious Dominican text, but is less convincing as an example of his beliefs when set against other evidence: the medical translations, which we know he almost certainly carried out as a friar, and his miracles.[13] The rest of this essay will project Duffin's approach back

---

[11] For some of these debates see *Locating Medical History: The Stories and their Meanings*, edited by Frank Huisman and John Harley Warner (Baltimore, 2004).

[12] Jacalyn Duffin, *Medical Miracles: Doctors, Saints and Healing in the Modern World* (New York, 2009).

[13] Iona McCleery, '*Multos ex medicinae arte curaverat, multos verbo et oratione*: curing in medieval Portuguese saints' lives', in *Signs, Wonders, Miracles: Representations of Divine Power in the Life of the Church*, edited by Kate

in time and explore where medical study of medieval healing miracles has got to today, and consider how it can move on in the future.

Medieval Miracles and Medical History

How should a medical historian start working with miracles? For some audiences, it is still an uphill battle to show that religion matters to medicine and vice versa. It is not enough to argue that the use of a healing plaster by a saint was an example of medical skill. The historian has to explain in great detail that the plaster used by Isabel of Aragon in the miracle described above was similar to those recommended by male surgeons and that domestic medical practices were integral to medieval healthcare.[14] The problem is that medical history has evolved in a separate sphere to religious or political history. Even the social history of medicine has had an identity crisis, falling awkwardly between medical sociology, medical humanities and social history.[15] The result is that non-medical historians sometimes miss the nuances of current research in medical history, and medical historians do not do enough to integrate their field into historical studies more broadly.[16] As a field, medical history has blossomed in the last twenty years. It is no longer just about medical manuscripts and university learning, although these things do not cease to be important, but includes

Cooper and Jeremy Gregory, Studies in Church History, 41 (Woodbridge, 2005), 192-202.

[14] Montserrat Cabré, 'Women or healers? Household practices and the categories of health care in late medieval Iberia', *Bulletin of the History of Medicine*, 82 (2008), 18-51.

[15] Roger Cooter, 'After death/after-"life": the social history of medicine in post-postmodernity', *Social History of Medicine*, 20 (2007), 441-64; Jonathan Toms, 'So what? A reply to Roger Cooter's "After death/after-'life': the social history of medicine in post-postmodernity"', *Social History of Medicine*, 22 (2009), 609-15; Brian Dolan, 'History, medical humanities and medical education', *Social History of Medicine*, 23 (2010), 393-405.

[16] Monica Green, 'Integrative medicine: incorporating medicine and health into the canon of medieval European history', *History Compass*, 7 (2009), 1218-45.

everything that shelters under the umbrella of medicine today. It therefore deserves more attention from beyond the field.[17]

Medical history is far removed from what it was when Ronald Finucane and Pierre-André Sigal started analysing miracles in the 1960s and 1970s, adopting a large-scale socio-statistical approach that has proved very influential.[18] Their approach appears quite different to that of Ernest Wickersheimer, a pioneering medical historian whose 1922 micro-study of the canonization process of Peter of Luxembourg (1387-1390) seems to be the earliest medico-historical analysis of any cult.[19] As Finucane pointed out in his historiographical overview of miracles, nineteenth- and early twentieth-century scholars such as Wickersheimer could see that miracles might be 'useful' for understanding the social context of medical practice.[20] Yet for C. Grant Loomis in 1940, in what seems to have been the first study of miracle cures in an academic medical history journal, miracles were curiosities 'for the student of folk-medicine'.[21] Writing in the same journal in 1986, nearly fifty years later, paediatrician Eleanora Gordon was more receptive to miracles as evidence for medieval childcare, but she still maintained that 'historians are appropriately sceptical about the historical validity of hagiographical literature'.[22] If we compare the attitudes of two

[17] For recent research see *Social History of Medicine*, 24 (2011), a special issue on the middle ages; *Between Text and Patient: The Medical Enterprise in Medieval and Early-Modern Europe*, edited by Florence Eliza Glaze and Brian K. Nance (Florence, 2011).

[18] Pierre-André Sigal, 'Maladie, pélerinage et guérison au XIIe siècle: les miracles de Saint Gibrien à Reims', *Annales*, 24 (1969), 1522-39; Pierre-André Sigal, *l'Homme et le miracle dans la France Médiévale (XIe-XIIe siècle)* (Paris, 1985). For Finucane, see note 9 above.

[19] Ernest Wickersheimer, 'Les guérisons miraculeuses du cardinal Pierre de Luxembourg, 1387-90', in *Comptes Rendus du Deuxième Congrès International de l'Histoire de la Médecine* (Évreux, 1922), 371-89. I have not been able to obtain a copy of this essay.

[20] Finucane, 'Use and abuse', 2-4.

[21] C. Grant Loomis, 'Hagiological healing', *Bulletin of the History of Medicine*, 8 (1940), 636-42.

[22] Eleanora C. Gordon, 'Child health in the middle ages as seen in the miracles of five English saints, AD 1150 - 1220', *Bulletin for the History of Medicine*, 60 (1986), 502. For a similar attitude, see Eleanora C. Gordon, 'Accidents among medieval children as seen from the miracles of six English saints and martyrs', *Medical History*, 35 (1991), 145-63.

historians working on healing miracles in another medical history journal eleven years apart we can see a further evolution in thought. Valerie Flint's important comparison of medicine, magic and religion in the early middle ages, published in 1989, warned that 'hagiographical material is full of traps for the historian and is hard to use; but it is full, also, of gold if only one can learn to sift it out'.[23] Flint felt obliged to justify her choice of source material quite carefully. In contrast, Clare Pilsworth did not feel she had to justify her subject at all in 2000. There was no sign of self-consciousness about her use of miracles; they sat easily within a special issue on early medieval medicine, demanding no less rigorous sifting than her complex archaeological, legal, chronicle and literary materials.[24]

More than a decade later, the landscape may be shifting again. Hilary Powell's very recent study of childbirth miracles begins by presenting these accounts as sources equivalent to obstetric and gynaecological texts, many of which as Green has shown have complex and contested authorship and transmission.[25] Yet she ends with an echo of Flint's caution from over twenty years earlier in the same journal, by saying 'miracle collections are a challenging source and should be read with caution and an acute sensitivity towards the actors governing their compilation and dissemination'.[26] This sensitivity of course applies to all sources, but it is not clear yet whether the renewed caution here towards miracles is widespread. In the specific context of childbirth, it may reflect a backlash against certain types of cultural relativism in gender studies.[27]

---

[23] Valerie Flint, 'The early medieval "medicus", the saint and the enchanter', *Social History of Medicine*, 2 (1989), 122.

[24] Clare Pilsworth, 'Medicine and hagiography in Italy, *c*. 800-*c*. 1000', *Social History of Medicine*, 13 (2000), 253-65.

[25] Monica Green, *Women's Healthcare in the Medieval West: Texts and Contexts* (Aldershot, 2000).

[26] Hilary Powell, 'The "miracle of childbirth": the portrayal of parturient women in medieval miracle narratives', *Social History of Medicine*, 25 (2012), 795-811, at 811.

[27] Iona McCleery, 'Medicine and disease: the female "patient" in medieval Europe', in *A Cultural History of Women in the Middle Ages*, edited by Kim Phillips (London, 2013), 85-104. See also the *Journal of the History of Sexuality*, 21 (2012), which is a special issue on medieval childbirth. The

It is easy to explain why there have been such differences in attitude over the decades. The impact on ecclesiastical history of the post-Second World War civil rights movement, the Annales school and the linguistic and cultural 'turns' is as obvious in hagiographical studies as in other fields. Miracles have long since proved themselves crucial for accessing minority groups such as children and the poor. The topoi of miracles ceased to be sifted through for nuggets of truth, but became embraced as significant sources for beliefs and attitudes in their own right.[28] What has been less acknowledged is how medicine itself changed out of all recognition over these same decades. It should not be surprising that there was greater criticism of miracles as historical sources during the technologicalization of healthcare that took place between the 1940s and 1980s. Historians from each part of the world understand the history of medicine and its debates to a very large extent in accordance with the systems of healthcare available in their own lifetime. As described above, medicine in the UK today has its own distinctive legal, political and financial character which affects the way the history of medicine is studied in the UK.[29]

Although it is easy enough to explain what has changed in the historiography of healing miracles, it is noteworthy how much more easily attitudes changed amongst scholars working on the period before 1000, mainly in Byzantine and Frankish studies.[30]

---

editor Margaret Cormack urges caution in the interpretation of all genres of source (201-07).

[28] Patrick J. Geary, *Living with the Dead in the Middle Ages* (Ithaca, 1994), 9-29; *The Miracles of Our Lady of Rocamadour*, edited and translated by Marcus Bull (Woodbridge, 1999); Sharon Farmer, *Surviving Poverty in Medieval Paris: Gender, Ideology and the Daily Lives of the Poor* (Ithaca and London, 2002); Michael E. Goodich, *Lives and Miracles of the Saints: Studies in Medieval Latin Hagiography* (Aldershot, 2004); Michael E. Goodich, '*Mirabilis Deus in sanctis suis*: social history and medieval miracles', in *Signs, Wonders, Miracles: Representations of Divine Power in the Life of the Church*, edited by Kate Cooper and Jeremy Gregory, Studies in Church History, 41 (Woodbridge, 2005), 135-56.

[29] For some reflection on how contemporary medicine affects historiography, see Flurin Condrau, 'The patient's view meets the clinical gaze', *Social History of Medicine*, 20 (2007), 525-40.

[30] Harry J. Magoulias, 'The lives of the saints as sources of data for the history of Byzantine medicine in the sixth and seventh centuries', *Byzantinische*

Other parts of central and southern Europe have been neglected for all periods. Early medieval medical historians like Clare Pilsworth and Peregrine Horden seem much more comfortable with miracles than late medievalists. The former group can incorporate hagiography more easily into the history of medicine because they have long been recognised as key narrative sources for all aspects of the early middle ages. Early-medievalists are often more interdisciplinary in their approaches, combining excellent skills in philology and manuscript studies with archaeology and theology. Late medievalists and early-modernists still seem to feel awkward about using miracles. These later scholars have a richer range of archival sources, more abundant medical sources, and the need to engage with modernists on issues like professionalization and secularism. For the fourteenth and fifteenth centuries, it therefore still tends to be the case that miracles are left to ecclesiastical historians. There are some notable exceptions: Michael McVaugh, Nancy Siraisi, Joseph Ziegler and Katherine Park all incorporate miracles into their social and cultural histories of late-medieval medicine.[31] Yet it seems that healing miracles still hold a different status as a source genre for those working on the period after 1000 compared to earlier. The later we go in the period of study, the more likely it is that healing miracles cease to be integral to the study of health and illness and become a completely separate field. This is why Duffin's study of modern miracles is so striking in its scope and approach, consciously taking methodologies developed originally by medievalists into the twentieth century and combining them

---

Zeitschrift, 57 (1964), 127-50; Peregrine Horden, 'Saints and doctors in the early Byzantine empire: the case of Theodore of Sykeon', in *The Church and Healing*, edited by William J. Sheils, Studies in Church History, 19 (Oxford, 1982), 9; Aline Rousselle, 'Du Sanctuaire au thaumaturge: la guérison en Gaule au IVe siècle', *Annales*, 31 (1976), 1085-1107; Michel Rouche, 'Miracles, maladies et psychologie de la foi à l'époque Carolingienne en Francie', in *Hagiographie: cultures et sociétés, IVe-XIIe siècles*, edited by Evelyne Patlagean and Pierre Riché (Paris, 1981), 319-37.

[31] Michael R. McVaugh, *Medicine Before the Plague: Practitioners and their Patients in the Crown of Aragon, 1285-1345* (Cambridge, 1993), 136-38, 142, 148n; Nancy Siraisi, *Medieval and Early Renaissance Medicine* (Chicago, 1990), 39-42, 153, 166; Katharine Park, 'The criminal and the saintly body: autopsy and dissection in Renaissance Italy', *Renaissance Quarterly*, 47 (1994), 1-33.

with her experience as a clinician and modern historian of medicine.³² It is this more integrated approach that we should be moving towards.

Some Portuguese Case Studies

In the rest of this essay, the aim is to explore some of the aforementioned debates in the context of three late medieval Portuguese cults. Portugal is an intriguing case study because one of the key reasons put forward for why healing miracles proliferated and became more medicalized from the late twelfth century does not seem to apply. It is usually argued that the establishment of papal canonization from the late twelfth century saw an increase in the quantity, sophistication and medicalization of healing miracles as proofs of sanctity.³³ Yet despite the existence of many flourishing miracle cults in Portugal, there were no formal processes (not even failed ones) until the early-modern period.³⁴ Most saints were only 'officially' recognised after the Counter-Reformation: Isabel of Aragon was canonized in 1625; Gil de Santarém was beatified in 1748.

Although some recent studies of saints' cults have downplayed the significance of canonization, on the whole historians still view the pope as the arbiter of sanctity.³⁵ Historians neglect regions and time periods where political and financial problems made it unlikely that there would ever be many, if any, papally recognised

---

³² Duffin acknowledges the influence of Ziegler and Park: Duffin, *Medical Miracles*, 8.

³³ André Vauchez, *Sainthood in the Later Middle Ages*, translated by Jean Birrell, 2nd edn (Cambridge, 2005), 61-84; Michael E. Goodich, *Miracles and Wonders: The Development of the Concept of Miracle, 1150-1350* (Aldershot, 2007), 68-99. For an alternative argument that healing miracles declined after the twelfth century, see the essay by Irina Metzler in this volume.

³⁴ Vauchez, *Sainthood*, 134, 270. An exception was Anthony of Padua/Lisbon (died 1231, canonized 1232), but Vauchez, *Sainthood*, 262, 271n, justifiably lists him as an Italian saint. Note that this neglect of hagiography extends across much of the Iberian Peninsula. See Anthony Lappin, *The Medieval Cult of Saint Dominic of Silos* (Leeds, 2002), ix.

³⁵ Aviad Kleinberg, 'Canonization without a canon', in *Procès de canonisation au moyen âge: Aspects juridiques et religieux*, edited by Gábor Klaniczay (Rome, 2004), 7-18; Sari Katajala-Peltomaa, 'Recent trends in the study of medieval canonizations', *History Compass*, 8 (2010), 1083-92.

saints. Yet the increasing importance of legal proofs of sanctity and the need therefore for medical prognosis could have developed separately from papal demands. In Portugal, mendicant interests may have produced the same effects. The question of why friars did not bother to send their documents to the pope is not an issue that can be explored here.[36] Not only does Portugal appear unusual in its saints' cults, it also seems not to fit classic models of the history of medicine. It had a single weak university and no discernible medical guilds. Hardly any medical manuscripts survive. Around eighty percent of physicians were Jews, theoretically expelled at the end of the fifteenth century. Yet we should beware concluding that late medieval Portugal was medically backward; it may be that it just does not fit the paradigms that historians have established for France, Italy or England.[37]

If Portugal is problematic in both its medical and its hagiographical profile, how can its healing cults be of use to a medical historian? What does 'medicine' mean in Portuguese miracles? Can we find only opposition between Christ and Galen, as Gil de Santarém allegedly stated, or is there something more to discover by combining different methods and approaches? First, it is important to introduce the three cults that will be used as case studies. What follows is an outline only; suggestions as to why these cults developed as they did come later. The cult of Gil de Santarém has already been referred to in this essay. There has been some debate over when it first developed, as the Latin *vitae* all date from the sixteenth century. The collection of miracles used in this study was completed in manuscript in *c.* 1543 as part of a renaissance dialogue, but not published until 1586 after the death of its author André de Resende, a celebrated Portuguese humanist. Most scholars accept Resende's claim that he used a three hundred-year

---

[36] Maria de Lurdes Rosa, 'A santidade no Portugal medieval: narrativas e trajectos de vida', *Lusitânia Sacra*, second series, 13-14 (2001-2002), 369-450; Maria Clara de Almeida Lucas, *Hagiografia medieval Portuguesa* (Lisbon, 1984); Mário Martins, 'Peregrinações e livros de milagres na nossa idade média', *Revista Portuguesa de História*, 5 (1951), 87-236.

[37] I explore this medical world in my monograph in progress: *Medicine and Community in Late Medieval Portugal (c. 1300-c. 1500)*.

old manuscript: the majority of the sixty-six posthumous healing miracles are set shortly after Gil's death in 1265.[38]

The second cult to be studied is that of Our Lady of the Olive Tree in Guimarães, a small town in northern Portugal. This cult sprang into existence in the mid-fourteenth century after the arrival of a holy cross caused a dry olive tree to revive, leading to cures attributed to the Virgin Mary. The clergy of the local collegiate church recorded the miracles and organised a series of processions around the town. All the forty-four healing miracles were originally recorded in 1342-43 by local notary Afonso Peres 'before the pestilence', but copied anew in 1351.[39] Afonso Peres presented his narratives in proper notarial style, supplying all the accounts with witnesses and dates. His miracle collection is the earliest to survive in the Portuguese vernacular, which might indicate that it was meant for a lay rather than a clerical audience, although it would be usual for a Portuguese notary to use the vernacular in this period. It may have already become the norm for miracles to be recorded in this way, although few earlier examples survive. It does not need to imply that Afonso Peres was influenced by papal criteria for canonization.[40]

The third cult is that of Bom Jesús or the Holy Name of Jesus, which inspired a collection of thirty-three miracles compiled in Portuguese in 1432 by André Dias, Benedictine monk, prolific author of theological works and bishop of the Greek diocese of

---

[38] André de Resende, *Aegidius Scallabitanus: um diálogo sobre Fr. Gil de Santarém*, edited by Virgínia Soares Pereira (Lisbon, 2000).

[39] Mário Martins, 'O livro de milagres de Nossa Senhora da Oliveira de Afonso Peres', *Revista de Guimarães*, 63 (1953), 5-54 (p. 28). See also Cristina Oliveira Fernandes, 'O livro dos milagres de Nossa Senhora de Oliveira de Guimarães', *Lusitania Sacra*, second series, 13-14 (2001-2002), 597-607; Cristina Oliveira Fernandes, *O Livro dos milagres de Nossa Senhora da Oliveira da Real Colegiada de Guimarães* (Guimarães, 2006).

[40] Earlier examples include an original notarial document in Portuguese recording two miracles presented as evidence at a Franciscan inquiry into the cult of Isabel of Aragon held shortly after her death in 1336. There is no evidence at all that these miracles were recorded for a formal canonization process and ultimately only one of them made it into her *vita*. See Pedro de Azevedo, 'Inquirição de 1336 sobre os milagres da Rainha D. Isabel', *Boletim da segunda classe da Academia das Sciências de Lisboa*, 3 (1910), 294-303; Iona McCleery, 'Isabel of Aragon (d. 1336): model queen or model saint?', *Journal of Ecclesiastical History*, 57 (2006), 668-92.

Megara. He attended the Councils of Constance (1414-18) and Basle-Ferrara (1431-37), dying in either 1437 or 1450-51, aged perhaps over a hundred. The Holy Name of Jesus was one of a number of Christocentric devotions that became fashionable in fifteenth-century Europe. At exactly the same time as Dias compiled his collection of miracles, the fiery preacher Bernardino of Siena was popularising the cult in Italy through his sermons, defending it against accusations of idolatrous heresy in 1426, 1431 and 1438. Dias less controversially responded to a plague epidemic in Lisbon in November 1432 by founding an altar and confraternity dedicated to Bom Jesús in the Dominican priory, preaching there to large audiences who subsequently experienced a series of cures using water blessed in the Holy Name. Promoting this cult in a Dominican priory might be explained by Dias's youthful entry into that order before becoming a Benedictine monk, but it is a little strange, especially as the Dominicans were strongly opposed to the cult in Italy.[41]

The Socio-Statistical Approach

It is possible to analyse healing miracles according to two key methodological approaches: the socio-statistical and the cultural. To start with the socio-statistical approach: there is something inherently countable about miracles. Even when a historian only has a dozen of them the temptation arises to calculate percentages of men, women and children, numbers of childbirths or cases of blindness. Since the time of Sigal and Finucane the socio-statistical approach has formed the bread-and-butter of hagiography and is still prominent as a starting point in most modern studies of medieval cults.[42] It is easy to apply to our Portuguese cases.

---

[41] Mário Martins, *Laudes e cantigas espirituais de Mestre André Dias (d. c. 1437)* (Negrelos, 1951), 283-98; António Domingues da Costa, *Mestre André Dias de Escobar: figura ecuménica do século XV* (Rome, 1967); Franco Mormando, *The Preacher's Demons: Bernardino of Siena and the Social Underworld of Early Renaissance Italy* (Chicago, 1999), 87-89, 103-05; Ephrem Longpré, 'Bernardin de Sienne et le nom de Jésus', *Archivum Franciscanum Historicum*, 28 (1935), 443-76; 29 (1936), 142-68.

[42] See most recently Anne E. Bailey, 'Wives, mothers and widows on pilgrimage: categories of "woman" recorded at English healing shrines in the high middle ages', *Journal of Medieval History*, 39 (2013), 197-219. This

The miracles of Our Lady of the Olive Tree in Guimarães record the cures of seventeen males (39%) and twenty-seven females (61%); a very high number, twenty-four (54%), were youths or children.[43] Just over half of the individuals (52%) had problems with vision (evenly distributed between the sexes) but there were eleven cases of possession (25%), all but two involving females. The range of ailments is quite narrowly biblical, but the number of females (including fourteen of the children and young people) is surprising since in many cults they often number little more than a third of cases.[44] The status of the recipients seems relatively lowly, although in many cases no information is provided; there are several people of artisanal status – a cobbler, a miller and a potter – as well as a monk, a notary and a squire. Higher status clergy and nobility were involved only in the processions. Most people came from the northern dioceses of Portugal (Braga and Porto). In the miracles of Bom Jesús in Lisbon, we encounter the more common ratio of twenty males (61%) to thirteen females (39%); seven (21%) were youths or children. They all appear to be local to Lisbon and a mixture of artisans (a carpenter, a cobbler, a tailor, a sailor, a rope-maker, a butcher and a scabbard-maker) and minor royal officials such as tax collectors and a porter. Apart from two clerics and a squire, there were no prominent participants. The range of ailments is more varied than in Guimarães – fevers, headaches, problems with feet, eyes, teeth, gout and sciatica – but the most striking cases are five that focus on pestilential symptoms. Plague miracles are very unusual in miracle collections.[45]

---

article begins with a statistical approach but then turns to a nuanced study of language and the lifecycle.

[43] My figures differ slightly from those in Fernandes, *Livro dos milagres*, 50-54, 61-62. In both the vernacular collections, a youth is consistently referred to as a *mancebo/manceba* and a child as *moço/moça*.

[44] In the cults analysed by Sigal, *L'Homme et le miracle*, 242, 259-61, 300-301 and Finucane, *Miracles and Pilgrims*, 143, 149, the proportion of female recipients is 20% to 40%. Explanations include the reduced likelihood of female injury or limited female access to monastic shrines.

[45] Nicole Archambaut, 'Healing options during the plague: survivor stories from a fourteenth-century canonization inquest', *Bulletin of the History of Medicine*, 85 (2011), 531-59.

In the miracles of Gil de Santarém there were forty-five males (68%) and twenty-one females (32%); of these twenty-two (33%) were youths or children.[46] Although only a third of the recipients of cures were female, women had easy access to Gil's tomb and relics, promoting the cult in 45% of cases. There was a wide range of injuries and ailments for both sexes, including eleven cases (16%) of traumatic injury, seven cases (11%) of fertility or childbirth-related problems and four (6%) cases of possession.[47] In thirty-three cases (50%) there were explicit references to medical practitioners, medical or surgical treatments and specialist diagnoses such as fistula, quinsy and hernia. The status of those cured varied widely from a prince with a fish bone in his throat through to royal courtiers, merchants, artisans and poor labourers such as a charcoal burner. They came from all over Portugal, but the majority were from within thirty to sixty miles of Santarém, a town about sixty miles up the River Tagus from Lisbon.

The socio-statistical approach is an essential start to any major study of saints' cults. Without a thorough knowledge of the people involved and the cures they received, no further analysis is possible. Yet there are problems with this approach which become apparent as soon as one tries to compare cults studied by different people. Each cult is studied according to a different agenda. For example, Sigal did not look for saintly specialisms in healing or break down his cures into fine enough sub-categories. Another problem is the tendency towards reductionism: reducing illness down to simplistic categories, as Finuncane and Sigal have both been accused of doing, obscures the many cases when recipients of miracle cures had multiple and recurring health problems.[48] Retrospective diagnosis –

---

[46] The Latin terms for these life stages are consistently *puer /puella* for 'child' and *adulescentulus /adulescens* for a male 'youth'. There is one case of *adulescens mulier*.

[47] Fifty-nine percent of the women did not have gynaecological or obstetric problems.

[48] See the critique of Finucane in Yarrow, *Saints and their Communities*, 10-11; and the implicit critique of both Sigal and Finucane in Irina Metzler, *Disability in Medieval Europe: Thinking about Physical Impairment in the High Middle Ages, c. 1100-c. 1400* (London, 2006), 216-85. These critiques also include Benedicta Ward, *Miracles and the Medieval Mind: Theory, Record and Event, 1000-1215*, rev. edn (Philadelphia, 1987).

using modern diagnoses to compile statistics or explaining away cures by referring to nutrition, psychosomatic illness or the placebo effect – has also come under fire in recent years.[49] It does not help us understand medieval experiences of illness and it completely side-steps the issue of religious belief.[50] For each of the Portuguese cults described above, we have to take into account the different time periods, places and scribal traditions, and we have to learn how to interpret nuances of language and gesture without assuming that they will be comparable to French or English experiences. Sensitivity towards the language of the body helps us to see that Gil de Santarém had an ears, nose and throat specialism.[51] Similarly, a close reading of the exorcism rituals reveals that the possession cases in Guimarães involved the ghosts of the deceased, a rare phenomenon in other parts of Europe.[52] The socio-statistical approach can provide us with a lot of useful data but it cannot help us interpret it on its own.

The Cultural Approach

Attention to language and ideas about the body brings us onto another major approach to hagiography. Careful cultural study of

[49] Andrew Cunningham, 'Identifying disease in the past: cutting the Gordian Knot', *Asclepio*, 54 (2002), 13-34; Jon Arrizabalaga, 'Problematizing retrospective diagnosis in the history of disease', *Asclepio*, 54 (2002), 51-70; Piers Mitchell, 'Retrospective diagnosis and the use of historical texts for investigating disease in the past', *Journal of International Palaeopathology*, 1 (2011), 81-88.

[50] For a much more nuanced study of medieval belief in 'magical' or 'miraculous' cures, see Matthew Milner, 'The physics of holy oats: vernacular knowledge, qualities, and remedy in fifteenth-century England', *Journal of Medieval and Early Modern Studies*, 43 (2013), 219-45.

[51] Twenty-four of Gil's cures (36%) were linked to the area between the gullet/neck and the ears, including fish bones in the throat, facial fistula, quinsy, scrofula and ear inflammation.

[52] These Portuguese cases are very different to the Castilian exorcisms analysed in Lappin, *Medieval Cult*, 131-69, who nevertheless provides some interesting analysis. On ghost possessions, see Éva Pócs, 'Possession phenomena, possession-systems: some east-central European examples', in *Communicating with the Spirits*, edited by Gábor Klaniczay and Éva Pócs (Budapest, 2005), 84-139; Nancy Caciola, 'Spirits seeking bodies: death, possession and communal memory in the middle ages', in *The Place of the Dead: Death and Remembrance in Late Medieval and Early Modern Europe*, edited by Bruce Gordon and Peter Marshall (Cambridge, 2000), 66-86.

symbols, constructions, rhetoric and discourse, gesture and emotion in miracles can help us move beyond typology and enable deeper understanding. There have been some excellent studies of saints' cults from this perspective but so far few medical historians have ventured down this path; striking examples are Peregrine Horden's interpretation of saints combating dragons as a response to disease and Irina Metzler's use of miracles in her study of disability and impairment.[53] Cultural historians of medicine have preferred to study the history of the body or childbirth rather than saintly cures.[54] Cultural historians of religion seem to prefer gender to illness.[55] There has been very little micro-historical work on healing cures to match Jean-Claude Schmitt's study of the cult of St Guinefort, the 'holy greyhound', over thirty years ago. His combination of theological, archival, literary, heraldic and archaeological evidence has yet to be matched.[56] Yet micro-historical study of individual cults (focusing on healing rather than other aspects of canonization processes or miracle collecting) seems to be the way forward; it was carried out by Lappin for the eleventh-century Castilian saint Dominic de Silos in 2002, urged by Goodich in 2005 and became the next step for Duffin whose innovative overview of modern miracles lacked specificity.[57] Nicole Archambeau's recent study of emotional responses to pestilence in the canonization process of Delphine de Puimichel in 1363 takes care not to diagnose retrospectively and provides plenty of

---

[53] Peregrine Horden, 'Disease, dragons and saints: the management of epidemics in the dark ages', in *Epidemics and Ideas: Essays on the Historical Perception of Pestilence*, edited by Terence Ranger and Paul Slack (Cambridge, 1992), 45-76; Metzler, *Disability*.

[54] For example, Katharine Park, *Secrets of Women: Gender, Generation and the Origins of Human Dissection* (New York, 2006).

[55] As can be seen in *Gender and Holiness*, edited by Riches and Salih; *Gendered Voices: Medieval Saints and their Interpreters*, edited by Catherine M. Mooney (Philadelphia, 1999). It is striking that there is a chapter on gender and sexuality in *A Companion to Middle English Hagiography*, edited by Sarah Salih (Cambridge, 2006), but not one on illness.

[56] Jean-Claude Schmitt, *The Holy Greyhound: Guinefort, Healer of Children since the Thirteenth Century*, translated by Martin Thom (Cambridge, 1983).

[57] Lappin, *Medieval Cult*; Goodich, '*Mirabilis Deus in sanctis suis*', 155-56; Jacalyn Duffin, *Medical Saints: Cosmas and Damian in a Post-Modern World* (Oxford, 2013).

contextual detail including the political background.[58] Laura Ackerman Smoller's work on the cult of St Vincent Ferrer and Marcia Kupfer's study of iconography at the pilgrimage centre of Saint-Aignan-sur-Cher, are also promising examples of what could be done. However, the latter is marred by the author's insistence on explaining all symptoms as ergotism.[59] At times cultural historians need to pay more careful attention to context and chronology; the approach can provide useful interpretations but sometimes not enough data to back them up.

To turn back to our Portuguese cults, some of the richness and the difficulties of the cultural approach can be seen in the three miracles selected for the appendix. They were deliberately chosen as representing the kind of motor problems that Sigal, Finucane and José Mattoso, author of the only study of health in Portuguese miracles, identified as typical in medieval miracles.[60] A contracted hand or limb, as in the miracle from Guimarães concerning the boy João, is a fairly common condition in miracles, too easily explained away as some kind of psycho-somatic illness. This is something that could be argued in the Guimarães cases where emotional conflicts may have led to illness in some cases: a girl objecting to her mother's choice of husband for her, an illness occurring shortly after marriage. Yet to boil these cures down to modern psychology is too limited. In Santarém, on the other hand, the child Benedict (see appendix) was expertly treated by surgeons who were not blamed for their failure to restore the function of the arm. The quantity of medical detail in this miracle obscures the emotional response of the mother. Like many other women in this collection, she went to Gil's tomb 'heartbroken' as a last resort when all else had failed. Even the most medicalized of cults cannot ignore emotions.

---

[58] Archambeau, 'Healing options'.

[59] Laura Ackerman Smoller, *The Saint and the Chopped-Up Baby: The Cult of Vincent Ferrer in Late Medieval and Early Modern Europe* (Ithaca, 2014); Marcia Kupfer, *The Art of Healing: Painting for the Sick and the Sinner in a Medieval Town* (Pennsylvania, 2003).

[60] José Mattoso, 'Saúde corporal e saúde mental na idade média Portuguesa', in his *Fragmentos de uma Composição Medieval*, 2nd edn (Lisbon, 1993), 233-52; Sigal, *L'Homme et le miracle*, 256-57; Finucane, *Miracles and Pilgrims*, 144-48.

Broken bones represent far greater problems of interpretation than do contracted limbs: either historians have to believe that the bones were actually broken and healed, or they have to cast aspersions over the diagnostic skills of the people involved.[61] A broken leg and hip as in the Bom Jesús miracle (see appendix) is not something easily explained away by the healing power of nature, since for normal physical function to return, the bones would have to have been set. This fracture constitutes what Mary Fissell has identified as a 'hard' illness as opposed to a 'soft' condition like possession; not meaning to denigrate this condition but rather to refer to its ease of cultural analysis. Not surprisingly there are not a lot of histories of broken bones.[62] Yet all these miracles are interesting for what they reveal about bodily function, expectations of normal movement and response to recovery. They tell us as much about healthiness as they do about illness. In line with Irina Metzler's essay in this volume, the emphasis at the end of the Bom Jésus miracle on getting back to work suggests what expectations might have been while labour was at a premium during successive plague epidemics and a period of intense expansion into North Africa and the Atlantic islands.[63]

Christ versus Galen in Portuguese Context

The last section of this essay will go back to the question raised in the first section: what was medicine in these three Portuguese cults? The cult of Gil de Santarém seems on the face of it to have an understanding of medicine similar to our narrow concept of professional practice and specialist treatments. In a case similar to the boy Benedict, with his paralysed arm, we hear of a boy called Pedro 'hit

---

[61] For similar problems to do with childbirth, see Margaret Cormack, 'Better off dead: approaches to medieval miracles', in *Sanctity in the North: Saints, Lives and Cults in Medieval Scandinavia*, edited by Thomas A. Dubois (Toronto, 2008), 334-52.

[62] Mary Fissell, 'Making meaning from the margins: the new cultural history of medicine', in *Locating Medical History: The Stories and their Meanings*, edited by Frank Huisman and John Harley Warner (Baltimore, 2004), 364-89. For a superb cultural analysis of a 'hard' condition (artherosclerosis), see Annemarie Mol, *The Body Multiple: Ontology in Medical Practice* (Durham, 2002).

[63] Metzler, 'Indiscriminate healing'.

on the head with such a great blow that the surgeon extracted eighteen bones and skull fragments, and cut various places of the skin in order to uncover and inspect the seams of the skull'.[64] The treatment would have been successful had the child not irritated the wound with his restlessness. In other cases we find operations for scrofula, the lancing of a suppurating abscess with a scalpel, cautery for a fistula, the application of bandages, fomentation of an abscess and fumigation of the ears. In most cases these procedures were carried out by people described as *medici* and usually given the title 'master', although the last example is something that Gil himself advised in a dream. He also repaired a hernia and drained an abscess in dreams.[65]

Despite these seemingly straightforward examples of what constituted medical practice, we also find less 'professional' activities. In one case a river boatman suffering from dropsy:

> had the skin around the pubic area and above the ankles cut nine times, and with his stomach ulcerated in many places, the work of Pedro Martins and Maria Martins and a certain Jew, who at that time was deemed very skilled in this kind of thing, it all availed to nothing.[66]

In this case also, the practitioners, even though female or Jewish, were not explicitly blamed for their failure to cure. Unusually, Gil scolded the boatman (in a vision) for spending money on physicians and surgeons, perhaps because his poverty did not justify such expenditure, but it implies that even those not deserving of the title 'master' were still practising medicine and surgery. Only once was a practitioner explicitly blamed for worsening a condition.[67] Instead it was usually assumed that the sick person would previously or even concurrently have sought medical help. This medical help often came from the Dominican friar-physicians themselves; people came to Santarém to seek medical aid from

---

[64] André de Resende, *Aegidius Scallabitanus*, 485.

[65] André de Resende, *Aegidius Scallabitanus*, 521, 586, 595. Dream-surgery can be found in many cults: see Finucane, *Miracles and Pilgrims*, 67-68.

[66] André de Resende, *Aegidius Scallabitanus*, 557.

[67] Master Martinho, 'then a well-known (nobilis) surgeon', examined a pustule 'with a very fine scalpel' but 'only succeeded in stirring it up and making it worse': André de Resende, *Aegidius Scallabitanus*, 494.

them, only visiting Gil's tomb as an after-thought. For example, the mother of a boy with a nosebleed took him to the priory 'to seek the advice of the friar-physicians (*fratres medici*) Andre and Bernardo'. They first prescribed some medication and then suggested she went to Gil's tomb.[68] Despite the pious words put in Gil's mouth by the compilers of the *Lives of the Brethren*, it is clear that even if Christ was more powerful than Galen, as he had to be within the context of a miracle collection, the friars in charge of the cult were not going to denigrate either themselves or other local practitioners. Since they were practising amongst the laity in defiance of contemporary Dominican bans on their doing so, their positive attitude towards medicine and surgery in these miracles must reflect an appreciation amongst the friars for the importance of medicine to their primary preaching mission.[69] In keeping with Duffin's findings for modern canonization processes, it was probably their expert medical prognosis that ensured these cures were viewed as miraculous.[70] The social range of people receiving cures reflects Dominican activity in an important fluvial port and frequent residence of the royal court in a country that was fairly recently still conquering land from the Muslims in the south. There were still significant Jewish and Muslim communities in the area and opportunities to engage with Islam in Spain and North Africa.[71] In order to understand the role of medicine in Gil's cult we should not therefore dwell too much on the medicalized terminology, some of which could actually date from the sixteenth century, and focus instead on the religious significance of medicine, a significance shared by all three cults.[72]

---

[68] André de Resende, *Aegidius Scallabitanus*, 505.

[69] Angela Montford, 'Dangers and disorders: the decline of the Dominican Frater Medicus', *Social History of Medicine*, 16 (2003), 169-91.

[70] Jacalyn Duffin, 'The doctor was surprised; or, how to diagnose a miracle', *Bulletin of the History of Medicine*, 81 (2007), 699-729.

[71] *S. Frei Gil de Santarém e a sua época*, edited by Jorge Custódio (Santarém, 1997).

[72] Remember that these miracles come from Resende's renaissance dialogue. A reference to the classical medical author Celsus, whose work was not rediscovered until the fifteenth century, was certainly a later addition: André de Resende, *Aegidius Scallabitanus*, 492.

Neither of the other cults would initially have attracted a medical historian. There are no references at all to any form of alternative healing in the Guimarães miracles, whether the illness was recent or 'from birth'. In Lisbon there is one reference to the failure of 'medicines' (*meezinhas*) and one mention of bloodletting.[73] Medical practitioners did not appear in either cult. The Guimarães miracles seem so old-fashioned by fourteenth-century standards – the number of biblical topoi and the ghostly possessions amongst other things – that one forgets to wonder why there were no references to medicine. Although no documented physicians have been found so far for fourteenth-century Guimarães, the eminent participants in the processions that were used to promote the miracles, such as the Archbishop of Braga and Count Pedro de Barcelos (the illegitimate son of a king), most certainly would have been familiar with physicians at court. Physicians appeared in other Portuguese miracle collections from the fourteenth century.[74] The decision to rely on communal testimony as proof that a miracle took place, rather than referring to medical evidence, must surely have been deliberate. These peculiar miracles should be set against a tense political background. The arrival of the cross that sparked off the cult may have been linked to memorialisation of the Battle of Salado in 1340, the last big set-piece battle between Christians and Muslims in the Iberian Reconquista.[75] There may also have been links to long-term conflict between the collegiate church in Guimarães and the Archbishop of Braga.[76] If we add to these political tensions the large numbers of women and children and interpret them as indications of inter-generational and familial conflict, it is possible to see the

---

[73] Martins, *Laudes e cantigas*, 289, 292.
[74] See McCleery, 'Curing', 195-96, and my monograph in progress, *Medicine and Community*.
[75] The existing fourteenth-century cross in the main square of Guimarães next to the collegiate church does indeed commemorate this battle. For discussion of how this battle was memorialized, see Bernardo Vasconcelos e Sousa, 'O sangue, a cruz e a coroa: memória do Salado em Portugal', *Penélope*, 2 (1989), 28-48; Solange Corbin, 'Fêtes Portugaises: commémoration de la victoire chrétienne de 1340 (Rio-Salado)', *Bulletin hispanique*, 49 (1947), 205-18.
[76] Fernandes, *Livro dos Milagres*, 29-38.

processions that resulted from the miracles as the primary healing events; the cures themselves were less significant than the communal processing around the town at regular intervals over several months. In addition, one wonders whether the decision to get Andre Peres's successor (did Peres die of plague?) to recopy the miracles several years later after the Black Death was another attempt at communal healing after further upheavals.[77] There is so little contemporary evidence for the effects of the Black Death in fourteenth-century Portugal, that tantalising glimpses like this are worth their weight in gold.

If we turn to Andre Dias's miracles in Lisbon, compiled also within a plague context, we again get a sense of communal healing processes, this time through Dias's own preaching. It is very significant that throughout his collection Dias repeatedly chose to describe the holy water blessed in Jesus' name as a *meezinha*, the same word he once used to describe earthly medication. In fact at times his miracles almost read like a series of medical case histories, all cured by the same patent remedy. Although there is no reference to turmoil as a result of plague, Dias does seem to have been concerned by the political context. His prologue refers to the political achievements of King João I (1385-1433) as miracles in themselves. João had successfully usurped the throne (although of course Dias did not refer to it as a usurpation), had fought and won wars against Castile, negotiated peace and then invaded North Africa in 1415. The healings are presented as further signs of divine favour. Yet there must have been some anxiety of what was going to happen to the new dynasty now that the king 'was in his old age and reaching the end of his life'.[78] It may be no accident that so many of the people mentioned in this collection were the artisans and lesser royal officials of Lisbon, the kind of people who had supported João I in his bid for the throne in 1383-85. If this were the target audience, it may even explain why Dias chose to promote

---

[77] The major study of Guimarães in the late middle ages does not analyse the miracle collection, but it does comment on the deaths of numerous notaries in this period, to the extent that notarial activity ground to a halt by the end of 1348; however, there appears to be no independent record of Peres. See Maria da Conceição Falcão Ferreira, *Guimarães: 'duas vilas, um só povo': estudo de história urbana (1250-1389)* (Braga, 2010), 440-41.

[78] Martins, *Laudes e Cantigas*, 283-84.

the cult of the Holy Name in a Dominican church; an altar in a church of his own Benedictine order would have limited the participation of people whom Dias hoped would remain supportive of João I's dynasty in the future.[79] Rather than merely restoring physical health, the purpose of this cult may have been to maintain political health.

Finally, to come back to Gil de Santarém's cures: for all their attention to medical detail, they were still profoundly religious and used similar healing metaphors to the other cults. In the case of Maria Gonçalves who had a horrible fistula on her face, applications of the earth from Gil's tomb 'worked more favourably and effectively than all the plasters, ointments and potions of physicians', including those of three friars who could only suggest removing her teeth.[80] In another case, Domingas Pires used earth and prayer to be healed of an abscess, pleading:

> with tears to the blessed man that, since in life he had been a physician not only of souls but also of bodies and had cured many through the art of medicine and through word and prayer, and now that he was powerful with God, he would deign to cure this his supplicant.[81]

What the Dominicans seem to be doing here in their miracle collection is using earthly medicine, both actual and metaphorical, to reinforce their religious message. Gil, both physician and healing saint, was an extraordinarily useful tool to disseminate the faith around Santarém and its environs. At one point, when asked during his lifetime why he anointed the eyes of a blind man rather than treating him medically, Gil answered that faith was stronger than art, comparing himself to Christ who also anointed the eyes of the blind 'against medical precepts' (*contra medicorum regulas*).[82] Although there is no mention of Galen, who might be said to

---

[79] Humberto Baquero Moreno, 'Reflexos da peste negra na Crise de 1383-85', *Bracara Augusta*, 37 (1983), 373-86; Joel Serrão, *O carácter social da revolução de 1383*, 6th edn (Lisbon, 1985); Valentino Viegas, 'Uma revolução pela independência nacional nos finais do século XIV', unpublished doctoral thesis (University of Lisbon, 1996).

[80] André de Resende, *Aegidius Scallabitanus*, 582.

[81] André de Resende, *Aegidius Scallabitanus*, 499.

[82] André de Resende, *Aegidius Scallabitanus*, 414-16. If Gil said this, he could have been referring to John 9: 1-12 or perhaps to Mark 8: 22-26.

represent 'medical precepts', this is a very close formulation to that in the *Lives of the Brethren*, a work that Resende did use in his compilation. Yet rather than opposition, this alternative version implies co-existing beliefs and values. By the early fourteenth century, learned surgeons such as Henri de Mondeville would be using the same biblical motif of anointing the eyes of the blind to identify Christ as a surgeon and themselves as divinely-inspired, quasi-priestly practitioners.[83]

To conclude: Jacalyn Duffin referred to modern medicine and religion as two intertwined belief systems. For medieval cults, it is useless to disentangle the two systems. The whole point of miracles is that they are about faith. If we try to disentangle healing miracles from the medical practices that they certainly do reveal, as so many scholars did in the past looking for competition between Christ and Galen, we are missing the point. Medicine in these miracles is a form of religion, hence the reason why friars continued to use it to make contact with their congregations. Religion can be a form of medicine in that it heals communities in unexpected ways. We need to be sensitive to our own attitudes towards both medicine and religion before we try to study medieval cults. There is much still to be done through careful combinations of social-statistical analysis and cultural methods as long as we pay attention to the contexts of both past and present.

---

[83] McCleery, 'Curing'; Simone C. Macdougall, 'The surgeon and the saints: Henri de Mondeville on divine healing', *Journal of Medieval History*, 26 (2000), 253-67; Ziegler, *Medicine and Religion*, 176-267.

Acknowledgements

The research in this essay was funded by the Wellcome Trust (grant number 076812). I would like to thank Louise Wilson and Matthew Mesley for inviting me to present a version of this paper at the 'Contextualizing Miracles' conference in Cambridge in April 2011.

Appendix

Gil de Santarém
The boy Benedict, son of Dona Mor de Guimarães who lived in Santarém outside the city walls near the church of the Holy Trinity, was watching a horse race when a horse, urged on too sharply and running wild, turned to the other side of the track, knocked him over, trampled him, and crushing his arm on the ground, broke it to pieces. Well, the labour of certain surgeons joined and consolidated the broken bones, but due to the severity of the damage to the nerves the hand was paralysed so that he could neither close his fist, nor bend his fingers, nor pick up anything in any way whatsoever. His mother was heartbroken because of this and went to the tomb of the holy man in supplication and, taking a little earth from there, bound it to her son's arm. From that moment he regained perfect health and was able to move his hand as he wanted; now closing it in a fist, then beginning to move his fingers, either contracting or extending them. He had completely recovered the use at will of his arm and his hand.[84]

Our Lady of the Olive Tree, Guimarães
On the same day [Sunday 2 February 1343], there was a miracle done on a little boy called João, said to live in the parish of São Martinho de Lagares, whose left hand and fingers were contracted. Having mercy on him, Holy Mary set him to rights and he opened his hand and fingers and closed the hand. He, and those who knew him from home, said there had never been a time when the hand had opened. That day, there were in town Count Pedro [of Barcelos, natural son of King Dinis], Archbishop Dom Gonçalo Pereira [of Braga] and many others in their company. The cantor,

---

[84] André de Resende, *Aegidius Scallabitanus*, 532.

clerics and choir canons, seeing these miracles [there were five that day] organised a procession. I, Afonso Peres, notary of Guimarães wrote this miracle. Witnesses: Gil Lourenço, Gil Peres, Martim Anes, notary; Vasco Domingues, almoxarife [tax inspector]; Bartolomeu Peres and others.[85]

Holy Name of Jesus (Bom Jesús)
This same Vasco Lourenço [a carpenter living near the church of St Nicholas] said that while his lad was riding a horse along the road, the horse stumbled and the boy had such a great fall that he immediately broke his right leg and his hip in such a way that he could not move from the place and had to be brought home. That night before he went to sleep, having great faith in and devotion to Bom Jesús, he drank the holy water in His Holy Name and washed the leg and hip with it and threw himself down to sleep. When he woke up he found his leg whole and the hip as well, as if it had never been broken or sickly. He got up straightaway the next morning and went to work as he had done before, thanks to Bom Jesús.[86]

---

[85] Martins, 'Livro de milagres de Nossa Senhora da Oliveira', 37.
[86] Martins, *Laudes e Cantigas*, 291.

INDISCRIMINATE HEALING MIRACLES IN DECLINE: HOW SOCIAL REALITIES AFFECT RELIGIOUS PERCEPTION

Irina Metzler

Narratives of miraculous healing abounded in both textual and visual sources of the earlier and high middle ages.[1] A particularly attractive iconographic, and chronologically rather late, example may be found in the detail of a predella from San Niccolò, Florence,[2] painted by Gentile da Fabriano in 1425, which shows groups of pilgrims with various physical and mental ailments approaching the shrine of St Nicholas of Bari: impaired and invalid pilgrims with their back to the viewer are making their way to the shrine, sometimes assisted by helpers, while a cured pilgrim carrying his now no longer needed crutches over his shoulder moves away from the shrine facing the viewer. But healing miracles, which had been so popular and numerous during the twelfth and thirteenth centuries, take a numerical nosedive from the fourteenth century onwards. This had already been noted by André Vauchez and Pierre-André Sigal among others, who have provided some interesting statistics on the topic.[3] During the early and high middle ages, saints 'appear primarily as miracle-workers, to whom one appealed to recover one's health'.[4] However, religiosity becomes more spiritualised in the course of the later middle ages,

---

[1] The chronological core of this essay concentrates on the twelfth and following centuries, although examples from earlier periods are cited as appropriate.

[2] Now located in Washington DC, National Gallery of Art.

[3] André Vauchez, *Sainthood in the Later Middle Ages*, translated by Jean Birrell (Cambridge, 1997); Pierre-André Sigal, *L'Homme et le miracle dans la France médiévale (X^e-XIIe siècle)* (Paris, 1985) and Pierre-André Sigal, 'Maladie, pèlerinage et guérison au XIIe siècle: les miracles de saint Gibrien à Rheims', *Annales*, 24.6 (1969), 1522-39.

[4] Vauchez, *Sainthood*, 466.

hence miracles become less 'practical' in the sense of curing people's physical ailments, instead becoming more rarefied and spiritual. Christianity as an organised religion had changed by the later middle ages from being a missionary faith that needed tools for conversion – and thaumaturgic miracles make excellent tools – to having become a firm part of daily life that required less practical reassurance. This argument was already made by Philip of Harvengt, a Praemonstratensian who died in 1183.[5] The 'practical' aspect of a miracle comes to take second place behind 'theological' miracles, such as visions, revelations or ecstatic experiences.[6] And even where miracles still retained a 'practical' aspect, this now tended to be focussed on deliverance and protection. The intriguing question is why should such a change have occurred.

By taking a closer look at an example of what 'miracle' meant for a late-medieval English writer one may attempt to answer this question. An anonymous English sermon, written between 1350 and 1450, discussed the healing miracle of a blind, mute and possessed man by Christ,[7] arguing that initially 'he was healed by the Lord so that he could speak and see'.[8] Taking two of Christ's miracles together, the sermon writer expands on the reasoning for such miracles: 'in one man three miracles were performed: a blind man sees, a mute man speaks, and a man possessed by a demon is made free. *On that occasion this happened in the flesh, but nowadays it happens in the conversion of believers* [my emphasis]'.[9] So originally

[5] In his life of St Waldetrude, Philip of Harvengt argued that since miracles were more effective in converting nonbelievers, they were widespread in the primitive church, but after 'the propagation of the faith, they had become infrequent': Michael Goodich, *Miracles and Wonders: The Development of the Concept of Miracle, 1150-1350* (Aldershot, 2007), 11; cf. Philip of Harvengt, 'Vita S. Waldetrudis', in *Monumenta poloniae historica*, volume 2 (Warsaw, 1864-1893), 1375.

[6] Vauchez, *Sainthood*, 468.

[7] Luke 11:14-28, although the same man is referred to in Matthew 12:22, where he is however described as mute and blind.

[8] The sermon is recorded in Cambridge: University Library, MS Kk.4.24, fols 292vb-294rb.

[9] Cambridge: University Library, MS Kk.4.24, fols 292vb-294rb. See also *Preaching in the Age of Chaucer: Selected Sermons in Translation*, translated by Siegried Wenzel (Washingon DC, 2008), 33. Similarly, the Augustinian preacher Jordan of Quedlinburg (*c.* 1300-1380) 'in his sermon for the second Sunday in Advent (based on Luke 7:22) regarded the blind who regain their

the purpose of this Gospel miracle was thaumaturgic, but by the sermon writer's own time it has a purely teleological function: it is primarily a means to faith and only secondarily an example of corporal healing. The writer explains further: 'after the demon has been driven out of them, they first see the light of faith, and then their tongues, which before had been silent, are loosened to praise God'.[10] Baptism and penance apparently fulfill similar functions as miracles, namely seeing the light of faith and speaking in praise of God. Where once Christ's healing miracle was 'in the flesh', it is now merely an adjunct to spiritual enlightenment.

Various cultural, social and economic changes from the thirteenth century onward were beginning to have an effect on perceptions of what constituted a 'proper' miracle. One factor revolved around medicalization. Just to briefly outline the argument here: in later medieval society overall one can speak of the concept of medicalization, in that there was a growth of public enthusiasm for bookish, learned, university medicine and greater public expectations of the medical profession; this is essentially Michael McVaugh's argument.[11] In a nutshell, medicalization leads to greater accessibility of (successful) medical treatment, thereby negating the need for seeking miracle cures, hence a decline in thaumaturgic miracles. But that is just one facet. Among other factors impinging on miracles one must consider also wider changes in later medieval culture. It is these I will focus on, most significantly relating to perceptions of who were the 'deserving' and 'needy' members of society, which in turn also influenced who was deemed a 'correct' recipient of a miracle.

Firstly, voluntary poverty (as practised by the mendicant orders) is culturally valued more highly and takes a higher ranking over involuntary poverty (as experienced by the unfortunate bottom

    sight as a metaphor for those who reach knowledge of God through understanding' (Goodich, *Miracles and Wonders*, 38); cf. Jordan of Quedlinburg, *Postillae de tempore* (Strasbourg, 1483), XV. *Sermo dominica secunda in Adventu*, fols 17r-18v; also Johann Baptist Schneyer, *Repertorium der lateinischen Sermones des Mittelalters für die Zeit von 1150-1350*, volume 3 (Münster, 1970-1980), 803.

[10] Wenzel, *Preaching in the Age of Chaucer*, 33.

[11] Michael M. McVaugh, *Medicine Before the Plague: Practitioners and their Patients in the Crown of Aragon, 1285-1345* (Cambridge, 1993).

rungs of medieval society), thereby affecting the social status of the poor, needy, invalid or disabled, whose position is reduced. Secondly, voluntary physical mortification, as practised by religious ascetics and mystics, is accorded higher value than the mundane suffering of the involuntarily disabled or sick: in short, if people who are held in high regard are actively and deliberately seeking out pain and illness as a gift from God, why should other people wish for their condition to be alleviated. This affects the religious status of disabled people.

Thirdly, in economic terms, the crises of the early- to mid-fourteenth century, coupled with rising numbers of the poor and beggars, narrows the amount of charity the rest of society is willing to provide. Prior to this period, isolated voices from the moralist camp could occasionally be heard lambasting the practice of indiscriminate charity, such as the canonist Rufinus of Bologna, who strongly advised against giving to those suspected of not deserving charity.[12] The thirteenth century appears to have been something of a pivotal era, when intellectuals, such as university masters, especially at Paris, and preachers, started spreading the message that the poor could be split into deserving and undeserving categories, with the additional accusation that the undeserving often fraudulently deceived the charitable donor.[13] Thereafter fear of 'fraudulent' beggars becomes common, and miracle cures of sick or disabled people become subsumed into the discourse of fraud. Stories surrounding fake cures are circulating and invalidating the 'real' healing miracles.

---

[12] Rufinus, *Summa ad dist.* 42 ante C.I, quoted in Brian Tierney, *Medieval Poor Law: A Sketch of Canonical Theory and its Application in England* (Berkeley and Los Angeles, 1959), 59.

[13] In the early thirteenth century Peter the Chanter set the tone by describing fraudulent beggars as changing their faces 'just like Proteus', so that acting (*histrionibus*) like truly sick people they deceived the donors: '*vultum sicut protea mutantes*'. Peter the Chanter, *Verbum abbreviatum*, c.48, *Patrologia Latina*, volume 205, col. 152, cited after Sharon Farmer, 'The beggar's body: intersections of gender and social status in high medieval Paris', in *Monks and Nuns, Saints and Outcasts: Religion in Medieval Society. Essays in Honor of Lester K. Little*, edited by Sharon Farmer and Barbara H. Rosenwein (Ithaca and London, 2000), 160, note 24.

Voluntary Poverty

Medieval understandings of poverty distinguished between voluntary poverty, which was understood as part of a religious vocation and was praised, and involuntary poverty, which was seen as resulting from a situation of social distress and increasingly came to be despised.[14] The phrase the 'poor of Christ' (*pauperes Christi*), meaning the religious poor, becomes frequent from the eleventh and twelfth centuries onwards.[15] Apostolic poverty was something to be imitated voluntarily by those people who according to their original status (one may here think of St Francis the wealthy merchant's son) were neither materially poor nor socially powerless. St Francis and his transformation from a rich man into a voluntary poor man had an enormous impact on the involuntarily poor, since while the concept of poverty as a spiritual discipline made it easier for the rich to gain salvation, the irony was that the poor *qua* involuntarily poor were precluded from the notion that their poverty could be used for spiritual means.[16] In the cogent interpretation by Sharon Farmer, the involuntary, economically

---

[14] However, Otto Gerhard Oexle has argued that the contrast between voluntary, religious poverty on the one hand, and involuntary, economic/social poverty on the other hand, has been exaggerated; furthermore poverty had come to be defined through manual labour in the high middle ages, so that in the case of St Elisabeth her aspirations to voluntary poverty included the real, involuntary poverty and physical work of the lower orders. Otto G. Oexle, 'Armut und Armenfürsorge um 1200: Ein Beitrag zum Verständnis der freiwilligen Armut bei Elisabeth von Thüringen', in *Sankt Elisabeth: Fürstin, Dienerin, Heilige. Aufsätze - Dokumentation - Katalog* (Sigmaringen, 1981), 79 and 92.

[15] Cf. Karl Bosl, 'Potens und Pauper: Begriffsgeschichtliche Studien zur gesellschaftlichen Differenzierung im frühen Mittelalter und zum "Pauperismus" des Hochmittelalters', in *Frühformen der Gesellschaft im mittelalterlichen Europa: Ausgewählte Beiträge zu einer Strukturanalyse der mittelalterlichen Welt* (Munich and Vienna, 1964), 121. On poverty and the mendicant orders in particular, see David Burr, *Olivi and Franciscan Poverty: The Origins of the Usus Pauper Controversy* (Philadelphia, 1989); also Hervaeus Natalis, *The Poverty of Christ and the Apostles*, translated by John D. Jones (Toronto, 1999).

[16] For a modern re-evaluation of St Francis and his propagation of voluntary poverty, see what Sharon Farmer reviewed as a 'deeply disturbing meditation on the meanings of poverty in western medieval Christianity', namely Kenneth Baxter Wolf, *The Poverty of Riches: St. Francis of Assisi Reconsidered* (Oxford, 2003).

poor can be associated with the flesh, while the voluntary, religious poor can be associated with the spirit.[17] Because the involuntary poor, who had not chosen to be poor, resented being in that state and desired change, in particular desired wealth, such desire, even if for just a modicum of possessions and money, endangered the spiritual health of the poor. According to Thomas Aquinas 'spiritual danger comes from poverty when it is not voluntary, because a man falls into many sins through the desire to get rich, which torments those who are involuntarily poor'.[18] Hence it was argued that it was better to give alms to the voluntary poor, since they did not fall into the sin of cupidity by desiring wealth, whereas the involuntary poor were consumed by desire. Already in the fourth century St Jerome had stated it was preferable to give alms to the voluntary poor than the involuntary ones 'among whose rags and bodily filth burning desire has domain'.[19] In the words of an eminent historian of poverty: 'the rule was that poverty could reach its apotheosis only as a spiritual value, while real, physical poverty, with its visible degrading effects, was perceived, both doctrinally and by society, as a humiliating state, depriving its victims of dignity and respect, relegating them to ... a life devoid of virtue'.[20] In a sense it is also preferable to receive a miracle when one is in a more virtuous state.

---

[17] 'Introduction', in *Monks and Nuns, Saints and Outcasts: Religion in Medieval Society. Essays in Honor of Lester K. Little*, edited by Sharon Farmer and Barbara H. Rosenwein (Ithaca and London, 2000), 13.

[18] Thomas Aquinas, *Summa theologiae*, 2a 2ae, quaest. 186, art. 3, resp. ad 2, volume 47 (Oxford, 1973), 108-11, cited by Sharon Farmer, 'Manual labor, begging, and conflicting gender expectations in thirteenth-century Paris', in *Gender and Difference in the Middle Ages*, edited by Sharon Farmer and Carol B. Pasternack (Minneapolis, 2003), 273.

[19] Jerome, 'Against Vigilantius', in *The Principal Works of St. Jerome*, translated by William H. Freemantle, The Nicene and Post-Nicene Fathers, 6 (Grand Rapids, Michigan, 1954), 422, cited by Farmer, 'Manual labor', 273.

[20] Bronislaw Geremek, *Poverty: A History* (Oxford, 1994), 31, cited by Livio Pestilli, 'Disabled bodies: the (mis)representation of the lame in antiquity and their reappearance in early Christian and medieval art', in *Roman Bodies: Antiquity to the Eighteenth Century*, edited by Andrew Hopkins and Maria Wyke (London, 2005), 96, note 43.

Voluntary Physical Mortification

As with the valorisation of religious poverty, the concept of saintliness defined by asceticism, physical deprivation and corporal mortification impacted on views of physical impairment. Already St Bartholomew of Farne (d. 1194) had held the maxim that 'we must inflict bad things onto our bodies if we want to lead them to the perfected glory of the soul'.[21] The cults developing around the Eucharist, Christ's body and Christ's wounds in the later middle ages contributed to this spiritualisation of religiosity, paradoxically thereby making later medieval religiosity more corporeal. From the twelfth and especially the thirteenth century onwards Christ's Passion came to be narrated, meditated upon, depicted and staged in the most concrete forms, so that countless faithful believers sought to emulate the sufferings of Christ using all conceivable means of self-torment, both imagined and physically enacted, a phenomenon for which historian Peter Dinzelbacher has aptly coined the term dolorism.[22] The pain that Christ had suffered had come to be regarded as the worst and greatest pain ever conceived, albeit a pain paling into insignificance in comparison with Christ's 'sorrow for perfidious humanity'.[23] Bodies of all sorts mattered more in the later middle ages than in the earlier period. Through the feast of Corpus Christi, the body of Christ, became notable and popular, female mystics experienced religious ecstasy through their bodies (especially through mutilations of their bodies), and the decaying body came to feature prominently on funerary monuments.[24] Self-inflicted pain and suffering were sometimes,

---

[21] 'Vita 9', Rolls Series, volume 75.1 (1882), 302, cited by Peter Dinzelbacher, 'Über die Körperlichkeit in der mittelalterlichen Frömmigkeit', in *Bild und Abbild vom Menschen im Mittelalter*, edited by Elisabeth Vavra, Schriftenreihe der Akademie Friesach, 6 (Klagenfurt, 1999), 52.

[22] Dinzelbacher, 'Über die Körperlichkeit', 60; Esther Cohen has also pointed this out: 'by the fourteenth century, physical suffering had become the landmark of living sanctity'. Esther Cohen, *The Modulated Scream: Pain in Late Medieval Culture* (Chicago, 2010), 27.

[23] Cohen, *The Modulated Scream*, 211.

[24] Cf. Caroline Walker Bynum, 'Warum das ganze Theater mit dem Körper? Die Sicht einer Mediävistin', *Historische Anthropologie*, 4.1 (1996), 14. For funerary monuments see especially Paul Binski, *Medieval Death: Ritual and Representation* (New York, 1996) and Pamela M. King, 'The cadaver tomb in

mainly among various mystics from the thirteenth century onwards, regarded as spiritually beneficial.[25] Caroline Walker Bynum noted that sickness and physical suffering were a highly gendered aspect of medieval mysticism:

> [F]or the late Middle Ages, there is clear evidence that behavior and occurrences that both we and medieval people see as 'illnesses' are less likely to be described as something 'to be cured' when they happen to women than when they happen to men. Women's illness was 'to be endured', not 'cured'. Patient suffering of disease was a major way of gaining sanctity for females but not for males.[26]

One wonders what medieval people then made of all those women who did seek out cures at the shrines of saints, more grist in the mill of those voices who trumpeted the moral inferiority of women, perhaps. For religious women who suffered in imitation of the sufferance of Christ, such pain, sickness and physical impairment were not disability as we would understand it, but means to achieve a spiritual goal. That very goal set them apart from 'ordinary' women who would rather not suffer. Active choice led some women, for instance Julian of Norwich, to pray for physical sickness. In Julian's case, she was only beginning to have visions of Christ's Passion once she contracted an illness which rendered her paralysed from the waist downwards.[27] The stigmata of Catherine of Siena (d. 1380) were, in contrast, not physically visible, but manifested themselves in strong inner pains felt by Catherine. 'The

---

England: novel manifestations of an old idea', *Church Monuments*, 5 (1990), 26-38.

[25] For an overview see Giles Constable, *Attitudes Toward Self-Inflicted Suffering in the Middle Ages* (Brookline, Massachusetts, 1982); Giles Constable, *Culture and Spirituality in Medieval Europe* (Aldershot, 1996), IX.

[26] Caroline Walker Bynum, *Holy Feast and Holy Fast: The Religious Significance of Food to Medieval Women* (Berkeley, 1987), 199.

[27] Julian of Norwich, *Revelations of Divine Love*, translated by Elizabeth Spearing (London, 1998), 44-45. A description of the pain behaviour of five women visionaries, Christina Mirabilis (1150-1224), Douceline of Digne (*c.* 1215-1274), Colette of Corbie (1381-1447), Margaretha Ebner (1291-1351) and Elisabeth Stagel of Töss (*c.* 1300-*c.* 1360), may be found in Cohen, *The Modulated Scream*, 121-28. Cohen further argued that 'practically all the holy women of the later middle ages, nuns as well as Beguines and laywomen, practised the self-infliction of pain and welcomed divinely inflicted sufferings'. Cohen, *The Modulated Scream*, 27.

stigmata were one aspect of the growing movement of physical identification with the suffering Christ; from the thirteenth century onwards it became the seal of sanctity, a sign of the outpouring of the Holy Spirit'.[28] As Jacques Le Goff has argued, such 'seals of sanctity' were only of concern to a small number of people with regard to the criteria of holiness, since religiosity in general and a sacred lifestyle were also factors, although female religious were especially prone to them.[29] Harsh asceticism, which included ritual self-mortification, was a feature especially of Dominican nunneries in the later middle ages, celebrated in the spiritual (auto)biographies of fourteenth-century nuns, with one aspect of relevance here being the 'therapeutic connotations of suffering'.[30]

Esther Cohen summarised the growing interest in (self-inflicted) pain in medieval culture, there was a morally beneficial element to it, and pain itself had a purpose:

> Late medieval pain culture was characterized by the multifarious ways in which pain was treated – even in fields of thought that we might consider irrelevant – and the tremendous positive significance identified in pain. Suffering was not to be dismissed, vanquished, or transcended: suffering was to be felt with an ever-deepening intensity[31]... Rather than being enslaved by a ferocious force that could dehumanize people, ascetics and self-inflictors became masters of pain, embracing it freely and using their sensations to reach new levels of spirituality.[32]

---

[28] Die Stigmen waren ein Aspekt der um sich greifenden Bewegung körperlicher Identifizierung mit dem leidenden Christus; seit dem 13. Jahrhundert wurde sie zum Siegel der Heiligkeit, ein Zeichen der Ausgießung des Heiligen Geistes. Jacques Le Goff and Nicolas Truong, *Die Geschichte des Körpers im Mittelalter*, translated by Renate Warttmann (Stuttgart, 2007), 63.

[29] Le Goff and Truong, *Die Geschichte*, 63.

[30] David F. Tinsley, *The Scourge and the Cross: Ascetic Mentalities of the Later Middle Ages* (Leuven, 2010), 21. One should note, however, that the definition of self-mortification did not extend to self-mutilation. To the modern mind there may be little between the two, but a medieval interpretation clearly differentiated them, so that mutilation, regarded as an infringement of divine creation of the body, was not entered into in religiously-motivated self-disciplines, although, in contrast, secular laws 'used mutilation as a standard punishment for specific offences'. Cohen, *The Modulated Scream*, 27.

[31] Cohen, *The Modulated Scream*, 3-4.

[32] Cohen, *The Modulated Scream*, 28.

Later medieval saints, mystics and flagellants were voluntarily marked physically in imitation of Christ's wounds. In contrast, real, living physically disabled people had received their impairment, wounds or mutilation involuntarily. As later medieval religion became more corporeal in this spiritualised sense, and especially as the suffering, mutilated, deformed or decaying body was interpreted through deeply religious sentiments, so conversely actual impaired people, who had not voluntarily mutilated themselves, but who had become disabled by chance, lost social, cultural and religious status. The voluntarily disabled, who were displaying religious mutilations or other bodily sufferings, needed to distance themselves from the common, unfortunate debilitated body. Healing miracles gave way to visions instead.

With the turning point in the thirteenth century, the saints themselves of the high and later middle ages reflected new attitudes to penance and contrition. To become a saint, one did not just have to cure people of intractable diseases, but what society expected of sainthood was now also an outward, demonstrative show of moral rectitude in the saintly persona.[33] Whereas in religious terms the early middle ages looked to the saints for the connection between God and humanity (through the process of intercession), a different order had emerged. The emphasis became ever more strongly placed on sacerdotal mediation between God and the normal believer, such as in the thirteenth-century *Rationale divinorum officiorum* of William Durandus.[34] This text described the rituals and semiotic system of late-medieval worship, down to the gestures the officiating priest should employ during the

---

[33] 'Just as the penitents changed, the saints changed. In addition to the traditional outward signs of sanctity, poverty and charity were increasingly demanded of them. Moral influence and apostleship counted for more than thaumaturgical or ascetic feats. The twelfth century had deepened their ideal of the mystical life': Le Goff, *Medieval Civilization 400-1500*, translated by Julia Barrow (Oxford, 1988), 350. Also Cohen, *The Modulated Scream*, 188: 'the charismatic presence of living saints, most of whom were said to have suffered a multitude of illnesses with great patience' bolstered the increasingly held view during the fourteenth and fifteenth centuries that 'illness was a salvific gift'.

[34] William Durandus, *Rationale divinorum officiorum*, edited by Anselme Davril and Timothy M. Thibodeau (Turnhout, 1995); cf. Miri Rubin, *Corpus Christi: The Eucharist in Late Medieval Culture* (Cambridge, 1991), 13.

ceremonies.³⁵ Increased emphasis placed on priestly intermediation and less placed on saints could also partly explain the decline in healing miracles, or were the saints simply becoming less accessible?

Involuntary Poverty and Disability

What worried later medieval people was the fake body, the body that pretends to be one thing but is in fact quite another: the theatrical delusion of the fraudulent beggar's artificially disabled body.³⁶ In *Piers Plowman* there were many such deceiving types: 'Langland knows them all, the guilers, lubbers, lollers, gadelings, false hermits, fobbes, faitors, bidders, leapers, lordains, lorels, mendinants, and their criminal associates the pissares, Robardsmen, Britonners, draw-latches and so on, creatures familiar enough in national and local ordinances and records'.³⁷ Late medieval society accused the poor of fraud, duplicity and faking, assuming that they begged even though they did not have an actual need for it. Begging had to be legitimated through need, and physical impairment could be regarded as one such legitimation. Many

---

³⁵ See *The Rationale divinorum officiorum of William Durand of Mende: A New Translation of the Prologue and Book One*, translated by Timothy M. Thibodeau (New York, 2007).

³⁶ Irina Metzler, 'Hermaphroditism in the western middle ages: physicians, lawyers and the intersexed person', in *Bodies of Knowledge: Cultural Interpretations of Illness and Medicine in Medieval Europe*, edited by Sally Crawford and Christina Lee (Oxford, 2010), 27-39.

³⁷ Geoffrey Shepherd, 'Poverty in *Piers Plowman*', in *Social Relations and Ideas: Essays in Honour of R. H. Hilton*, edited by Trevor H. Aston, Peter R. Coss, Christopher Dyer and Joan Thirsk (Cambridge, 1983), 173. But the character of Piers the ploughman, trying to discern between rightful and fraudulent alms-seekers, learns in the course of 'B' passus VI 'that he is not in a position to determine who is deserving or not ... all beggars ... are answerable to God individually. The onus is on the receiver'. Anne M. Scott, *Piers Plowman and the Poor* (Dublin, 2004), 109. On the material and spiritual economies in Piers Plowman see Roger A. Ladd, *Antimercantilism in Late Medieval English Literature* (Basingstoke, 2010). On the terminology used of fraudulent beggars, cf. Kellie Robertson, *Keeping Paradise: Labor and Language in Late Medieval Britain* (Basingstoke, 2004). On beggars, vagabonds and other non-settled marginal types in general in England, cf. *The Book of Vagabonds and Beggars*, edited by David B. Thomas (London, 1932); Jean J. Jusserand, *English Wayfaring Life in the Middle Ages*, translated by Lucy Toulmin Smith (London, 1888). More general is Jose Cubero, *Histoire du vagabondage du Moyen Age à nos Jours* (Paris, 1998).

depictions of the poor in fifteenth-century art therefore show the 'type' of the disabled, mainly the orthopedically impaired, beggar.[38] By the high middle ages the notion of indiscriminate charity was becoming refined. High medieval canonical theory tried to make ethical differences: only the 'just', the 'honest' and the 'shameful' poor were to receive charity. The decretists pondered the question of whether one should give charity indiscriminately, as St John Chrysostom had demanded, or whether to restrict charity to certain sub-groups of the poor, namely those who were deemed to be truly needy.[39] In such a way the giving of alms came to be connected more closely with exhortations to make oneself useful.[40] The notion of *utilitas* became more important, as expressed in the New Testament verse 'who does not work shall not eat'.[41] The categorisation of persons according to their ability to work (whence begging forbidden) or inability (whence begging allowed) constituted a paradigmatic underpinning of the discourse pertaining to concepts of deserving and undeserving poor.[42] In short, to that degree by which the value of work increased, the status of beggars decreased.[43]

In a case associated with the miracles of St Louis, 'the mother of a crippled girl believed that "God would be more favourable to them" if they lived by their own labour while they waited at Louis

---

[38] Robert Jütte, too, observed this trend. He added that for the sixteenth century the pauper 'was no longer characterized by physical deformities but was designated by begging gesture and a pathetic condition. This change reflects a new attitude to the poor. It was no longer a physical handicap that denoted a beggar, but something less concrete, less tangible: a gesture, a way of behaving, in short the physical and moral condition'. Robert Jütte, *Poverty and Deviance in Early Modern Europe* (Cambridge, 1994), 14.

[39] On this topic see Tierney, *Medieval Poor Law*, 55-60.

[40] Arnold Angenendt, *Geschichte der Religiosität im Mittelalter* (Darmstadt, 1997), 595.

[41] 2 Thessalonians 3:10.

[42] On poverty and the increased value placed on work cf. K. Bosl, 'Armut, Arbeit, Emanzipation', in *Beiträge zur Wirtschafts- und Sozialgeschichte des Mittelalters: Festschrift für Herbert Helbig* (Cologne and Vienna, 1976), 128 ff.

[43] In dem Maße, wie der Wert der Arbeit stieg, sank das Ansehen der Bettler. Frank Meier, *Gaukler, Dirnen, Rattenfänger: Außenseiter im Mittelalter* (Ostfildern, 2005), 39.

IX's tomb for a cure, and thus she did not want alms to be given to her daughter'.[44] Hence even the lower strata of urban society had subsumed the elite intellectual (clerical) discourse on the intrinsic value of labour that was coming to be propounded from the latter part of the thirteenth century onwards.[45] Being able to perform physical, manual work was valued long before the so-called Protestant work ethic. In the case of one relatively minor, localised saint, the point about the 'suggestive construction of a polarized, laboring body' is clearly made.[46] This statement is made in relation to St Walstan, originally an East Anglian noble (975-1016), with a subsequent shrine at Bawburgh, Norfolk, whose cult became especially popular during the fifteenth century, in effect becoming the patron saint of East Anglian agricultural labourers. What is of interest in St Walstan's *Vita* is the emphasis of miracles on the cure of impairments as a means to re-enable work. As 'specialist' for agricultural workers, whom he healed of any infirmity or bodily disability that prevented their labour, St Walstan exemplified the importance of being capable of earning one's livelihood.[47] In the fifteenth-century cult the most poignant miracle narrated in the collection includes a carter who was crushed by a laden cart and was so eager to return to work once cured that he did not even tarry

[44] Nolebant quod daretur ei elemosina, pro eo quod, sibi videbatur quod, si de suo labore hic [Louis's tomb] viveret cum filia sua predicta, magis esset propitius sibi Deus. 'Fragments de l'enquête faite à Saint-Denis en 1282 en vue de la canonisation de Saint Louis', edited by H.-François Delaborde, *Mémoires de la Société de l'Histoire de Paris et de l'Ile de France*, 23 (1896), 49, cited by Farmer, 'Manual labor', 277 and 287, note 55.

[45] The miracles of St Louis were written by Guillaume de St Pathus, one-time confessor to Louis's wife Queen Marguerite. To place the work ethics propounded here in a local, Parisian context, it is worth pointing out that the 'champion of work', William of St Amour, a near-contemporary master at the university, preached assiduously against the mendicants because they falsely lived off charity, while accepting that certain groups of people who were incapable of working, such as the very young or the very old and the sick, were deserving of charity. See Miri Rubin, *Charity and Community in Medieval Cambridge* (Cambridge, 1987), 73.

[46] Kellie Robertson, *The Laborer's Two Bodies: Literary and Legal Productions in Britain, 1350-1500* (Basingstoke, 2006), 32.

[47] Robertson, *The Laborer's Two Bodies*, 32; cf. *Nova legenda Anglie: As Collected by John Tynemouth, John Capgrave and Others, and First Printed, with New Lives, by Wynkyn de Worde*, edited by Carl Horstmann, volume 2 (Oxford, 1901), 412-15.

at the saint's shrine but rushed back to his village.[48] 'The usual charisma associated with saintly bodies here gets a contemporary colouring, allowing the injured worker to return to ... productive work as soon as possible'.[49]

In 1406 William Taylor, a Wycliffite reformer, preached a sermon on the themes of poverty, charity and work. In his text he proposed an extreme work ethic that contained elements of the sort of thinking behind the rapid return to work notions in St Walstan's miracles. Taylor alluded to the gospel healing miracles of Christ[50] and proposed that the miracles were not just about healing for the sake of it (or even to enable greater faith), but expressly so that these impaired 'clamorous beggeris' who 'would sit at gates and beside ways, and cry and beg' should no longer be reliant on alms.[51] Christ was allegedly motivated by a loathing of begging as much as by spiritual reasons, and performed these miracles to enable the disabled to earn their living through work: 'and in token that Christ loathed such begging, he healed such men not only in soul but also in body, that they might get what they need by their bodily labour'.[52] William Taylor valorised and elevated work as a virtue in itself, and even as a 'cure' for disability, generating the astonishing argument that Christ healed the sick first and foremost so that they could be put to work.

But the beggar's body, especially the disabled beggar's body, also came to be devalued, something to be hidden, and no longer to be publicly exhibited. Various late medieval begging laws required that

---

[48] For an account of this and other miracles in the English Life of the saint, cf. Montague R. James, 'Lives of St Walstan', *Norfolk Archaeology*, 19 (1917), 264.

[49] Robertson, *The Laborer's Two Bodies*, 36.

[50] Namely thaumaturgic miracles at Mark 10:46, Luke 18:35 and John 9:8.

[51] Weren nedid to sitte at ʒatis and biside weies, and crye and begge. 'The Sermon of William Taylor', in *Two Wycliffite Texts*, edited by Anne Hudson, Early English Text Society, original series, 301 (Oxford, 1993), 19, cited by Kate Crassons, '"The workman is worth his mede": poverty, labor, and charity in the sermon of William Taylor', in *The Middle Ages at Work*, edited by Kellie Robertson and Michael Uebel (Basingstoke, 2004), 79.

[52] And in tokenynge þat Crist loþide sich begging, he heelide siche men not oonly in soule but also in body, þat þei myʒten gete þat hem nedide bi her bodily labour. 'The Sermon of William Taylor', cited by Crassons, 'The workman is worth his mede', 79.

sick or disabled beggars covered themselves up, beggars were not to annoy the good citizens with the smell and sight of their disgusting wounds and infirmities, especially those with contagious diseases or severe physical impairments.[53] Even in the narrative of the thirteenth-century miracles of St Louis, the sight of a severely disabled person is something that contemporaries did not exactly welcome: Amelot of Chambly was so afflicted by her impairment, her body bent so that she could only crawl around St Denis, her head just held above the ground, which caused the children of the town to flee in horror when they saw her coming.[54] Therefore physical blemish or impairment had become something shameful that must be hidden, while conversely being the justifying factor for legitimate begging. With regard to their appearance, both their dirty, torn clothes and their physical condition, giving off a disagreeable odour and covered in pustulating sores, the begging poor person is sometimes described as *abiectus*, literally as abject, in the sources.[55] A graphic representation of the abjection of the poor beggar, both physically and metaphorically, can be found in a painting by Hieronymus Bosch of St Bavo distributing alms.[56] The saint, portrayed as noble, immaculately dressed and groomed, reaches into his purse to give money to an elderly woman (a widow, perhaps) carrying an infant on her shoulder while in the foreground

---

[53] Cologne begging laws; see Frank Meier, *Gaukler, Dirnen, Rattenfänger: Aussenseiter im Mittelalter* (Ostfildern, 2005), 37. Alle, die mit Krankheiten behaftet vor den Kirchen sitzen oder auf der Straße ihre widerlichen Wunden und Gebrechen zeigen, sollen diese verdecken, damit die wohlgesetzten Bürger (gude lude) durch den Geruch und Anblick nicht belästigt werden. Cited in Franz Irsigler and Arnold Lassotta, *Bettler und Gaukler, Dirnen und Henker: Außenseiter in einer mittelalterlichen Stadt. Köln 1300-1600* (Munich, 1989), 26. For similar laws also at Regensburg, probably influenced by nearby Nuremberg, see Artur Dirmeier, 'Armenfürsorge, Totengedenken und Machtpolitik im mittelalterlichen Regensburg: Vom hospitale pauperum zum Almosenamt', in *Regensburg im Mittelalter: Beiträge zur Stadtgeschichte vom frühen Mittelalter bis zum Beginn der Neuzeit*, edited by Martin Angerer (Regensburg, 1995), 231.

[54] Sharon Farmer, *Surviving Poverty in Medieval Paris: Gender, Ideology, and the Daily Lives of the Poor* (Ithaca and London, 2002), 157.

[55] Michel Mollat, *Die Armen im Mittelalter*, translated by Ursula Irsigler (Munich, 1987), 11.

[56] Detail of the right wing of the 'Last Judgment', painted *c.* 1485-1500, now in Vienna, Akademie der Bildenden Künste.

a second small child stretches out its hands. In the background however, lurking out from behind the saint's cloak, sits a physically deformed beggar, holding up his twisted right arm while in front of him, on a piece of cloth, he is displaying an amputated and nearly mummified foot. The imagery is not just grotesque and abject, but also ambiguous: is this really the beggar's own foot, in which case he is one of the unfortunates deserving of St Bavo's charity, or is this a fake and the beggar is of the fraudulent type, undeserving and hence disregarded by the saint's charity?

The problem of physical appearance can also be found in the theme of the lame person who is miraculously healed against their will. In the *vitae* of St Martin of Tours, starting with the so-called Pseudo-Odon version dating to the turn of the eleventh to twelfth centuries, can be found stories relating to the translation of the saint's relics from Auxerre to Tours. Two lame men (variously referred to as *paralitici* in the Latin text, *kontret* in the twelfth-century rhymed *vita*, and *contrefaictz* in the fifteenth-century version) are terrified at the thought of being healed by the imminent miracle; one says to the other:

> Until now we lived in peaceful leisure. Nobody disturbs us, all have compassion with us. We only have to do as we like. In short, we spend our days in comfort. Should we be made well again through a miracle, then we would have to occupy ourselves with physical work to which we are not accustomed. We could no longer live from alms.[57]

---

[57] German text cited in Bronislaw Geremek, *Geschichte der Armut: Elend und Barmherzigkeit in Europa*, translated by Friedrich Griese (Munich and Zurich, 1988), 64. On the literary topos of the blind man and his guide and/or blind man and lame companion see Gustave Cohen, 'La scène de l'aveugle et de son valet dans le théâtre français du moyen age', *Romania*, volume 41 (1912), 346 ff; also Gustave Cohen, 'Le thème de l'aveugle et du paralytique dans la littérature française', in *Mélanges offerts à M. Emile Picot*, volume 2 (Paris, 1913), 393; André de la Vigne, *Moralité de l'aveugle et du boiteux* (Paris, 1831), xi; for the topos in a fabliau 'De trois aveugles de Compiegne', in *Recueil général et complet des fabliaux des XIIIe et XIVe Siècles*, edited by Anatole de Montaiglon and Gaston Raynaud, volume 1 (Paris, 1872), 70 ff. Farmer, 'The beggar's body', 159, note 19, gives the date of the text cited above, *De reversione beati Martini a burgundia tractatus*, as probably written between 1137 and 1156. The Latin text is cited by Farmer after André Salmon, *Supplément aux chroniques de Touraine* (Tours, 1856), 52: 'ecce frater, sub molli otio vivimus ... hoc autem totum nobis vindicat

Because life lived off alms is so convenient, the two lame men decide to flee before the impending miracle might occur. In their haste they grab their crutches, with which they used to beg, fling them over their shoulders and run away: in this fashion the miracle does after all take place. The topos is repeated in the *Exempla* of Jacques de Vitry and in the *Golden Legend* in the variant of a blind and a lame man, then picked up in *Pèlerinage de la vie humaine* by Guillaume de Deguilville in the 1330s in connection with the sin of Avarice.[58] Avarice is here described as an allegorical figure, surrounded by false images produced by her, namely Treachery and Deceivance. Once Avarice has tampered with the real, old images in churches, she visits all the fraudulent beggars in the land and has them pretend to be crippled and maimed, 'or deaf and dumb'.[59] These false disabled then come before one of the idols, itself a false image, made by Avarice, and cry out to be made well again. The third falsehood in this series is now a fake miracle as well. Michael Camille said of the hunchback and cripple kneeling before the false image in an illumination accompanying the text of *Pèlerinage*: 'the two cripples are also figures meant to elicit not sympathy but censure, since they are 'professionals', like those in the *exempla* of the two lazy beggars ... who vainly try to avoid the relics of St Martin so they may not be healed and lose their alms'.[60] We are back to the notion of physical impairment as the uppermost of a sliding scale of moral and anatomical defects that push the needy person ever downward. In the later middle ages, being poor and disabled is the prime cause for despondency leading on to sins of desire, envy and hopelessness.

   infirmitas haec qua jacemus; quae si curata fuerit, quod absit, necessario nobis incumbet labor manuum insolitus'.
[58] Thomas F. Crane, *The Exempla of Jacques de Vitry* (London, 1890), 112: 52 and 182; Jacobus de Voragine, *The Golden Legend: Readings on the Saints*, translated by William Granger Ryan, volume 2 (Princeton, 1993), 300.
[59] *The Pilgremage of þe Lyfe of þe Manhode: Translated Anonymously into Prose from the First Recension of Guillaume de Deguilville's 'Le Pélerinage de la Vie Humaine'*, edited by Avril Henry, Early English Text Society, original series (Oxford, 1985), 128, cited in Michael Camille, *The Gothic Idol: Ideology and Image-Making in Medieval Art* (Cambridge, 1989), 270.
[60] Camille, *The Gothic Idol*, 271, referring to the fourteenth-century copy in Paris: Bibliothèque Nationale, MS fr. 829 (Guillaume de Deguileville's *Pèlerinage de la vie humaine*: second recension), fol. 92v.

With the ambiguity and censure surrounding the physical appearance of (dis)abled beggars, later medieval sentiments concerning charity in the widest sense were changing. With the invention of indulgences, which began to increase in popularity from around 1230, individuals could care for their souls in a more professional way, so that instead of relying on the good will of a grateful beggar to pray for the donor's soul a person could enter into a transaction with the church's 'Treasury of Merits'. Thus Lester K. Little paraphrased a thirteenth-century Dominican writer's explanation of the system of indulgences: 'for a cash payment the penitent person could get credit against his penitential debt from the store of supplemental merit and good works on deposit there from the lives of Christ, Mary, and the saints'.[61] Charitable giving did of course continue in the later middle ages, such as bequests in wills, payments to the poor in return for attendance at one's funeral, and donations to specialised – not general – hospitals and almshouses, but these were all aspects of charity that were strongly tied in with direct, specific inter-personal relationships. The older style of indiscriminate, anonymous, even random doling out of charity was by the later period being supplanted by carefully thought out schemes of support for narrowly defined sets of individuals, the deserving poor, since it was their prayers that one bought. One may extend this notion of the commodification of grace even further, and ask: why give money to dirty, smelly and offensive beggars in the hope they will pray for your soul in humble gratitude, when you can have priests say proper masses in the refined setting of your own private chapel, making a powerful architectural statement concerning your wealth and influence at the same time? The contractual but relatively informal arrangement between the giver of alms and the recipient, who was to pray for the soul of the donor, may have been weaker in the later middle ages with the advent of chantry priests and chantry chapels from the thirteenth century onwards and especially during the fourteenth century.[62]

---

[61] Lester K. Little, *Religious Poverty and the Profit Economy in Medieval Europe* (London, 1978), 201.

[62] On chantry chapels see Simon Roffey, *The Medieval Chantry Chapel: An Archaeology* (Woodbridge, 2007); Simon Roffey, *Chantry Chapels and*

Chantries and associated chapels were designed to hear masses to ease the soul of the departed through purgatory. Therefore prior to the twelfth-century 'invention' of purgatory, famously described by Jacques Le Goff, chantries would have been a nonsensical aberration in religious terms.[63] From the late medieval period many examples in English cathedrals and parish churches survive for the delectation of enthusiastic art historians and tourist visitors. Chantries represented incorporations of priests saying masses for the soul of the departed, the staff so to speak, while chantry chapels denoted the architectural embodiment of the same incorporations. Together, chantries and chantry chapels 'professionalised' the economics of prayer. As D'Avray has shown, beginning with the thirteenth-century preaching manuals, the use of 'market-place vocabulary' and commercial imagery entered religious dialogue and texts.[64] In extension of this metaphor, it is suggested that the increased popularity of chantries and chantry chapels supplanted the need for the anonymous mass of the poor to pray for the souls of charitable donors. Individual poor persons, singled out for deserving status in bequests by some donors, such as the almsmen of God's House at Ewelme,[65] were under contractual obligation to pray for their benefactor's soul, but this does not detract from the main argument that the wider practice of indiscriminate giving of the earlier middle ages was being supplanted by more specific, defined and proscribed charity. Since a priest was only permitted to say one single mass per day, chantries required extra staffing if more than one mass was to be heard, and therefore ate up additional

---

Medieval Strategies for the Afterlife (Stroud, 2008); George H. Cook, *Mediaeval Chantries and Chantry Chapels* (London, 1963); Marie-Helene Rousseau, *Saving the Souls of Medieval London: Perpetual Chantries at St Paul's Cathedral, c. 1200-1548* (Aldershot, 2011); *The Medieval Chantry in England*, edited by Julian Luxford and John McNeill (Leeds and London, 2012).

[63] Jacques Le Goff, *The Birth of Purgatory*, translated by Arthur Goldhammer (Aldershot, 1990).

[64] David L. D'Avray, *The Preaching of the Friars: Sermons Diffused from Paris before 1300* (Oxford, 1985), 208-16.

[65] John A. A. Goodall, *God's House at Ewelme: Life, Devotion and Architecture in a Fifteenth-Century Almshouse* (Aldershot, 2001). I am grateful to the peer reviewer for drawing my attention to this statutory obligation of the residents.

funds that might otherwise have been given to the poor. This point was already made by medieval criticism of the 'waste' of money on fancy architecture and other material endowments, found in the popular tract *Dives and Pauper*:

> Me thynkith that it were betere to geuyn the monye to the pore folc, to the blynde and to the lame wose soulys God boughte so dere, than to spendyn it in solempnyte and pride and makynge of heye chyrchis, in riche vestimentys, ... for God is nought holpyn therby and the pore folc myghte be holpyn therby wol mychil [much].[66]

This is a truly materialistic assessment: keep material wealth for this world, and separate from the spiritual. How popular chantries were can be seen in late fifteenth-century Bristol, where among 18 parish churches could be found 120 temporary and 20 permanent chantries.[67] The exact correlation between the rise in popularity of the chantry chapel and the decline in direct material assistance given to the poor by private donors still needs to be assessed, but it is a startling coincidence that the hugely popular late medieval endowment of chantries occurs at the same period in time when the poor in general and beggars in particular came to be regarded as somewhat suspect.

The theses presented here are very much work in progress and aim to cover a lot of ground. Nevertheless some conclusions are in order to try and wrap up the evidence presented so far. Firstly, medicalization means greater availability of physicians, better trained physicians, and probably more effective medicine, which plays some role in demoting thaumaturgic miracle as a method of healing. Secondly, Christianity as an organised religion has by the

---

[66] *Dives and Pauper*, edited by P. Heath Barnum, Early English Text Society, original series, 275, volume 1, part 1 (Oxford, 1976), 189-90.

[67] Martyn Whittock, *A Brief History of Life in the Middle Ages* (London, 2009), 84. Extreme architectural expression of the demarcation between professional (the Mass said by a priest) and amateur (the prayers said by a grateful beggar) may be found in the so-called 'caged' chantries that started appearing in England during the fourteenth century (cf. unpublished paper 'Chantry chapels: building for death', given by Linda Monckton, English Heritage, at Leeds IMC, July 2008). The boundary between these two worlds is materially presented in the 'cage' surrounding the chantry, while the physical screen keeps out undesirables. Hence concern for the afterlife becomes a more private affair, conversely at the same time as outward expression of such concern becomes more public.

high middle ages taken firm hold in central and western Europe, so that these areas no longer need internal missionary activities. The thaumaturgic saint is no longer as valuable as a vehicle for conversion as s/he previously was. This is an observation nevertheless leaving open the question: do thaumaturgic miracles retain greater popularity in certain regions, like the Hispanic peninsula (where miracle working saints were useful for the conversion of the reconquered infidel), or in Scandinavia (which still experienced ongoing internal mission)? Thirdly, the expression of religiosity has changed, so that by the later middle ages voluntary poverty, as practised by the mendicant orders, and voluntary corporal mortification, as practised by mystics, ascetics and the 'new' saints, is valorised to the detriment of involuntary material poverty and disability. This causes, fourthly, an interiorisation of medieval religiosity within the sphere of private devotion as well as an almost 'hysterical' outward expression of religious mass-movements which run side by side in the later middle ages: 'the increase in the number of chantries, of processions, of fraternities, of pilgrimages, the inflation of devotional and edificatory literature, the expansion of clerical drama, the excessive cult of relics – that denotes late medieval piety in its emphasis on the quantitative and visible'.[68] Therefore, charity becomes more discriminating, fraudulence worries both donors and theologians, hence people have to prove they are worthy or 'needy', and the same applies to expectations of miracle: greater demarcation of the 'deserving' of both charity and/or miracle becomes the order of the day.

So we may ask the question, who then is the ideal recipient of a later medieval healing miracle? A modest person who is not fraudulently but genuinely disabled, meaning crippled, blind, deaf or dumb, who is incapable of working but does not beg aggressively, who has tried everything they can in this world first (that is, tried medical cures, sought the material help of family, friends or neighbours) before turning to otherwordly aid, and who,

---

[68] Die Zunahme der Meßstiftungen, der Prozessionen, der Bruderschaften, der Wallfahrten, das Anschwellen der Andachts- und Erbauungsliteratur, der Ausbau der geistlichen Spiele, die Übersteigerung im Reliquienwesen – das kennzeichnet die spätmittelalterliche Frömmigkeit in der Betonung des Quantitativen und Äußerlichen. Edith Ennen, *Die europäische Stadt des Mittelalters* (Göttingen, 1987), 253.

most importantly, does not expect a healing miracle. To paraphrase a modern educational protest slogan, in the earlier middle ages a healing miracle was a right not a privilege, but in the later period it became a privilege not a right. With the later medieval commodification of the means of grace, thaumaturgic miracles have become rationed and scarcer. Thus the ideal protagonist of a miracle toward the later medieval period is no longer the sick or disabled person seeking healing, but the morally virtuous person whose status of cultural evaluation according to ethical principles takes primacy over their status of corporal condition.

ST EDMUND OF EAST ANGLIA: 'MARTIR, MAYDE AND KYNGE', AND MIDWIFE?[1]

Rebecca Pinner

An Antiphon for a Queen

In January 1245, Eleanor of Provence (*c.* 1223-91), queen of Henry III (1207-72), was in labour with her fourth child. Mindful of the perils of childbirth, her husband had one thousand candles lit around the shrine of Thomas Becket at Canterbury and a further thousand in the church of St Augustine's in the same city.[2] Henry also instructed his clerks to chant an antiphon over his wife in order to speed her safe delivery. The success of this latter measure was joyfully recounted by the king in a letter to Henry of Rushbrooke (1235-48), abbot of the great Benedictine Suffolk house of Bury St Edmunds:

> Know that on Monday after the feast of St Hilary [16 January 1245], when our beloved consort Eleanor, our Queen, was labouring in the pains of childbirth, we had the antiphon of St Edmund chanted for her, and when the aforesaid prayer was not yet finished, the bearer of this recent letter, our valet [Stephen de Salines, told us that she had] ... borne us a son. So that you may have the greater joy from this news we have arranged for it to be told to you by Stephen himself. And know that, as you requested us if you remember, we are having our son named Edmund.[3]

---

[1] I would like to thank my thesis examiners, Katherine Lewis and Margit Thøfner, for encouraging me to further explore the miraculous episode upon which this chapter is based.

[2] *Calendar of the Liberate Rolls Preserved in the Public Record Office, Volume 2, Henry III AD 1240-45*, edited by William Henry Stevenson and Cyril Thomas Flower (London, 1930), 275.

[3] Sciatis quod die Lunae proxima post festum sancti Hilarii, laborante dilecta consorte nostra Aelianora regina nostra tristitia pariendi, fecimus pro ea psallere antiphonam de sancto Edmundo, et nondum completa oratione sequente praesentium lator Stephanus Salines valettus noster ad nos veniens

Henry's choice of saints is also not surprising: by the mid-thirteenth century Becket was arguably the pre-eminent saint in medieval England and the king's devotion to St Edmund is well attested.[4] As a royal saint, Edmund would be an appropriate guardian for a royal baby. The offering of votive objects, especially candles, at the shrine or image of a saint was common practice by those seeking assistance.[5] However, Henry's specific method of securing Edmund's assistance through the chanting of the antiphon over his wife is far less usual and raises a number of intriguing questions regarding the perceived nature of saintly intervention.

The Antiphon

The nature of the antiphon itself may offer some insight. Although the letter from the King fails to specify which antiphon was sung for his queen, it is likely to have been one of the most celebrated plainchant items associated with the abbey at Bury, four antiphons which formed part of the Office for St Edmund: *Ave rex gentis Anglorum*, *O purpurea martyrum gemma*, *Gaudes honore gemino* and *Princeps et pater patriae*.[6]

---

nuntiavit nobis quod praedicta regina nobis filium produxit in lucem sponsum ... Et sciatis quod sicut nos ipsi rogastis, si memoriter retinetis, faciemus ad ipsum filium nostrum, Edmundum nuncupari. *Chronicle of Bury St Edmunds, 1212-1301*, edited and translated by Antonia Gransden (London, 1964), 13. See also Margaret J. Howell, 'The Children of Henry III and Eleanor of Provence', in *Thirteenth-Century England IV: Proceedings of the Newcastle upon Tyne Conference 1991*, edited by Peter R. Coss and Simon D. Lloyd (Woodbridge, 1992), 63.

[4] For Henry III's devotion to St Edmund see Antonia Gransden, *A History of the Abbey of Bury St Edmund's 1182-1256* (Woodbridge, 2007), 245-48 and Antonia Gransden, 'The Abbey of Bury St Edmunds and national politics in the reigns of King John and Henry III', in *Monastic Studies: The Continuity of Tradition*, edited by Judith Loades, volume 2 (Bangor, 1991), 67-86.

[5] Ben Nilson, *Cathedral Shrines of Medieval England* (Woodbridge, 1998), 99-105.

[6] Music for the Office of St Edmund is printed in *Antiphonale Sarisburiense: A Reproduction in Facsimile of a Manuscript of the Thirteenth Century*, edited by Walter H. Frere (Farnborough, 1966). See also Rodney M. Thomson, 'The Music for the Office of St Edmund, King and Martyr', *Music and Letters*, 65 (1984), 189-93. See also Lisa Colton, 'Music and identity in medieval Bury St Edmunds', in *St Edmund, King and Martyr: Changing Images of a Medieval Saint*, edited by Anthony Bale (Woodbridge, 2009), 87-110.

These antiphons for first Vespers appear for the first time in the well-known *libellus* made at and for Bury *c.* 1125, now New York, Pierpont Morgan Library, MS 736, renowned for its set of full-page miniatures depicting the life, death and posthumous miracles of St Edmund, also contains a version of the earliest *Vita* of St Edmund by Abbo of Flerury (*c.* 945-1004), an anonymous *Vita et Miracula*, and Lessons and music for the Translation (20 April), *Passio* and Mass of St Edmund. The antiphons have no known textual source which has led Thomson to identify them with four antiphons composed a generation earlier by a monastic visitor to the abbey.[7] In *De miraculis Sancti Eadmundi*, the first collection of Edmund's miracles composed at Bury in the 1090s, the author Hermann notes that during his visit '*temporibus regis Willelmi prioris*' Abbot Warner (also known as Garnerius or Garnier) of Rebais (fl. 1105-1133) composed four antiphons in honour of St Edmund, thus dating them to before 1087.[8] Of these the *Ave rex gentis Anglorum* encapsulates the spirit of Edmund's multivalent saintly identity which the Bury monks worked so hard to promote in the decades following the Norman Conquest: Edmund is invoked as both regional patron and a universal intercessor and his power and compassion are equally praised:

> Hail, O King of the people of Anglia,
>
> Warrior of the Sovereign of angels!
>
> O Edmund, flower among martyrs,
>
> Like the rose or the lily,
>
> Intercede before God

---

[7] Thomson, 'Music', 192.

[8] Temporibus regis Willelmi prioris, venit ad abbatiam pretiosi martyris [Eadmundi] Warnerius Francigena quidam abbas Resbacensis, homo quidem religiosorum morum, sed etiam pollens dignitate litterarum, cum dulci modulatione neumarum. Is denique susceptus illuc officiosissime ... composita quattuor antiphonarum cantilena suavi ad honorem sancti, sic de die in diem ad ipsius amorem cœpit accendi, ut promereretur a Baldwino patre de pignoribus sancti recipere, quibus martyr in exteras regiones posset venerari, veneratus etiam circumquaque virtutibus notificari. '*Hermann archdiaconi liber de miraculis Sancti Eadmundi*', in *Memorials of St Edmund's Abbey*, edited by Thomas Arnold, volume 1, Rolls Series (London, 1890), 69-70.

For the salvation of your faithful flock.

Lord, open my lips,

And my mouth will announce your praise.[9]

In the context of childbirth the request for the Lord to open the lips of the one singing, or in this case hearing, the antiphon may have had a particular gynaecological resonance.

Furthermore, the *Ave rex* antiphon was widely disseminated and its popularity endured throughout the middle ages; in addition to the Pierpont Morgan MS it also appears in an antiphoner made for secular use in England in the second half of the twelfth century and in another *libellus* of unknown English provenance from the early 1200s.[10] Four motets and carols from fourteenth- and fifteenth-century Bury echo the phraseology of the antiphon.[11] The fifteenth-century *vita* of St Edmund composed by the Bury monk John Lydgate (*c.* 1370-*c.* 1451) also includes an exhortation for any whom 'to seynt Edmund haue deuocion/ With hool herte and dew reuerence/ Seyn this anteph[o]ne and this orison' which the poet recounts was 'write and registred afforn his hooly shrine', in order to be granted an indulgence of two hundred days.[12] In addition, the fifteenth-century tracery lights in the northwest nave window of St Edmund's church, Taverham (Norfolk) contain six demi-figures of angels wearing diadems and ermine tippets, four of whom survive, and who each bear an inscribed scroll with a verse from the *Ave rex* antiphon.[13] Antiquarian Francis Blomefield also records the

---

[9] Ave rex gentis Anglorum/ Miles Regis angelorum/ O Eadmunde flos martyrum,/ Velut rosa vel lilium/ Funde preces ad Dominum/ Pro salute fidelium./ Domine labia mea aperies/ Et os meum annuntibat laudem tuam. Cited in Thomson, 'Music', 192. The implications for the role of the antiphon in the construction of Edmund's saintly identity are discussed by Colton in 'Music and identity', 89-95.

[10] Stockholm: Rijksarkivet, Kammerarkivet Cod. Fragm. Ant. 203 and Oxford: Bodleian Library, MS Digby 109. Both are discussed by Thomson, 'Music', 190.

[11] See Colton, 'Music and Identity', 90-91.

[12] John Lydgate, *The Lives of Ss Edmund and Fremund and the Extra Miracles of St Edmund*, edited by Anthony Bale and Anthony S. G. Edwards (Heidelberg, 2009), Prologue, 73-80.

[13] David King, 'An antiphon to St Edmund in Taverham church', *Norfolk Archaeology*, 35 (1977), 387-91.

antiphon written on the now-lost chancel screen in Fundenhall church (Norfolk).[14] Further evidence of the propagation of the antiphon may be found in a number of medieval lead pseudo-coins found in St Mary's Church, Bury St Edmunds, which bear its opening words.[15] It is likely these were a form of pilgrim souvenir intended to remind devotees of the indulgence gained by visiting the shrine. Therefore the imagery of the text itself, along with the enduring cultural significance of the *Ave rex*, makes a compelling case for this being the antiphon chanted over Queen Eleanor on that cold January in 1245.

St Edmund

Nevertheless, the reasoning behind the choice of St Edmund as saintly midwife requires further interrogation. The saint after whom the safely-delivered baby was named was a favourite of successive monarchs and until the fourteenth century a national patron. An erstwhile ruler of the Anglo-Saxon kingdom of East Anglia who met his death at the hands of invading Vikings in 869, Edmund also enjoyed an enduring regional identity and a reputation as a chaste and devout martyr as well as a potent miracle-worker; between the 980s and the early sixteenth century four major collections of Edmund's miracles were compiled at Bury and numerous other accounts were incorporated into, or appended to, at least eight versions of his *Vita*.[16] As evident in the tripartite epithet 'martir, mayde and kynge', coined by Lydgate, Edmund's saintly identity was complex.[17] However, it was not as a patron of pregnancy or childbirth that Edmund was most frequently invoked. Indeed, the birth of this royal prince appears to be the only known example of Edmund being called upon to intercede in such

---

[14] Francis Blomefield, *An Essay towards a Topographical History of the County of Norfolk*, volume 5 (Fersfield, 1806), 174.

[15] Samuel Tymms, *A Historie of the Church of St Marie Bury St Edmunds* (Bury St Edmunds and London, 1845), 62-67.

[16] Rebecca Pinner, 'St Edmund, King and Martyr: Constructing his Sanctity in Medieval East Anglia', unpublished doctoral thesis (University of East Anglia, 2011), 61-173.

[17] Lydgate, *Lives of Ss Edmund and Fremund*. The tripartite formulation is first used in the Prologue, l. 56 and repeated frequently thereafter.

circumstances. This is particularly striking given the number and variety of miracles otherwise recorded.[18] It is possible that Henry's devotion to Edmund led to his invocation, or that the Bury monks saw an opportunity to capitalise on his preference by suggesting Edmund as a suitable candidate; Henry's allusion to the convent's request that the royal baby should be named after their saintly patron suggests that the forthcoming birth had at least been previously discussed.

Popular Devotion?

A further, and potentially more productive, alternative is that the absence of childbirth miracles within the *vitae* and *miraculae* authored at Bury suggests that Henry was responding to a version of Edmund's saintly identity which did not depend solely on the official authorised cult for its validity. This inevitably invokes the discourse of 'popular' devotion which in recent decades has come to prominence in scholarship of medieval religion. As an area of scholarly enquiry, popular religion has suffered from a tendency by some to over-emphasise a perceived distinction between high and low culture and to seek out only the non-official or even pagan. In the context of the study of medieval miracle narratives within the discourse of popular religion, great emphasis is placed on episodes which appear to preserve older, sometimes ancient, folk beliefs or manifest elements of pre-Christian practices within authorised Christian culture. Whilst these elements are undoubtedly present in some cases, in others it has resulted in over-simplification and the seemingly wilful over-looking of more complex and often more illuminating instances where different traditions merge.

'Popular religion' is a complicated term which defies precise definition, but which is sometimes understood to mark a distinction between learned and elite religion and the religion of the less-learned masses. As Simon Yarrow notes elsewhere in this volume, the notion of 'elite and popular religion' has continued to 'exercise' historians, citing a relatively recent volume of *Studies in Church History*, published in 2006 which, although aiming to

---

[18] See Pinner, *St Edmund, King and Martyr*, 356-62 for graphical comparison of the range of Edmund's miracles from the tenth to the fifteenth centuries.

unpick the elite-popular binary, Yarrow in fact believes 'confirmed the enduring afterlife of two-tier tradition'.[19] Some of the difficulties arising from this definition are readily apparent. In his important study of religious culture in England between 1050-1250 Carl Watkins sets out to challenge many of the assumptions about religious belief, such as the extent to which it is possible to divide people into discrete types, the possibility of defining 'learned' and 'unlearned' and distinguishing who belonged in each category, noting the reductive binaries often produced by assuming a correlation between patterns of belief and the social groupings of believers. He cites, for example, the case of monks and the aristocracy, noting that aristocratic families 'supplied the cloisters with recruits, were bound to them by the frequent exchange of gifts for prayers, and celebrated association with the life of renunciation because it seemed so valuable to the sinner in the world', concluding that 'monk and warrior were not marooned on either side of a cultural divide'.[20] In the context of the miracle under consideration, for example, most would probably agree that Henry III is not best described as low or unlearned. Furthermore, in the context of saints' cults, popular devotion would normally suggest the spontaneous development of beliefs or practices independently from the authorised cult. However, in the case of St Edmund the situation appears more complex. Whilst Edmund is not explicitly presented in the official cult as a patron of childbirth, reading this episode in the context of other aspects of his saintly identity render this association intelligible.

This paper therefore argues for a more nuanced reading of the miracle in question, advocating an interdisciplinary approach which accommodates sources too often isolated from each other by the imposition of disciplinary boundaries: 'official' miracle narratives, the symbolic and discursive significance of Edmund's physical remains, and practices such as the Bury St Edmunds white bull fertility ritual which elide easy categorisation. This line of enquiry

---

[19] Simon Yarrow, chapter 2 of this volume, 41, discussing *Elite and Popular Religion*, edited by Kate Cooper and Jeremy Gregory, Studies in Church History, 42 (Woodbridge, 2006).

[20] Carl S. Watkins, *History and the Supernatural in Medieval England* (Cambridge, 2007), 5-6.

allows a reappraisal of an historiographical tendency to privilege the monastic perspective in the construction of saintly identity and demonstrates the benefits of incorporating sources from the geographical and ideological cultic periphery.

Miracles and Childbirth: The Broader Context

Firstly, although it has been well-established elsewhere, it is worth reiterating that whilst the childbed miracle is unique within Edmund's saintly repertoire this is far from the case with other saints.[21] Henry's attempts to secure saintly protection for his wife and child at this perilous time are far from unique; indeed, Henry himself took similar precautions during the birth of a number of his other children.[22] The perils of childbirth were well attested in the middle ages, both by practical experience and in texts belonging to the *molestiae nuptuarium* (the perils of marriage) genre whose authors extolled the virtues and benefits of the religious life as opposed to the distractions and dangers, both spiritual and physical, of wedlock. Descriptions of childbirth provided particularly compelling examples of the dangers of the secular life, as seen in a letter written by Osbert of Clare (d. *c.* 1158), the twelfth-century prior of Westminster. Apparently at her request, Osbert writes to encourage Ida, niece of Queen Adeliza (*c.* 1103-1151), second wife of Henry I of England (*c.* 1068-1135), to remain true to her vows as a nun, praising the virginal life she has chosen and offering the 'burdens of pregnancy' as a vividly grim alternative:

> When a mother conceives earthly offspring she changes the condition of her entire nature and transfers into another the quality she had first displayed. Her countenance becomes pale and the brightness of the eyes is hollowed by thick darkness: the veins around the temples appear livid and the face, liable to ugliness, grows pale, and the colour, made dark by transient mutability, flees: the skin draws back wrinkles on the face and the roundness of the fingers diminishes on the hands: the swelling womb of the pregnant one is distended, and the organs

---

[21] Hilary Powell, '"The miracle of childbirth": the portrayal of parturient women in medieval miracle narratives', *Social History of Medicine*, 25.4 (2012), 795-811.

[22] Howell, 'The Children of Henry III', 57-72, 61-63.

burdened within are dispersed. These are the annoyances that earthly nuptials produce; these are the burdens that disturb daughters of Eve giving birth. Further, if any queen or empress or countess obtains the honour of her name in worldly majesty, in her conception she incurs the aversion of anguish no less than a poor little woman, nor does she, laden with gems and gold, either conceive or give birth in a palace in a different way than a resourceless and ragged woman in a hut. All conceive in sin, all give birth in sorrow; the trouble of Eve weighs down all, the sadness of the mother surrounds all.[23]

Although pre- and post-natal risks were certainly exacerbated by poor diet and hygiene, and therefore more pronounced amongst the lower echelons of society, Osbert, presumably to appeal directly to the high-born recipient of his epistle, reiterates that the dangers of childbirth were shared by all women, including the Queen of England.[24] Furthermore, as pregnancy was a threat to both the physical and spiritual health of the woman, divine protection was especially desirable.

Like Henry III, many expectant parents sought advice and assistance during the various stages of pregnancy and birth. Examination and treatment of pregnant and labouring women was

[23] Cum terrestrem parens concipit sobolem totius naturae suae mutat consuetudinem et in alteram transmigrat quam prius extiterat qualitatem. pallida facies eius efficitur et oculorum claritas densa caligine concavatur: apparent venae circa tempora lividae et pallescit vultus deformitate obnoxius et aufugit color decidua mutabilitate fuscatus: pellicula rugas in facie contrahit et rotunditas digitorum in manibus tabescit: uterus intumescens impregnantis distenditur, et viscera intrinsecus gravidata dissipantur. haec sunt taedia quae terrestres nuptiae generant; haec sunt onera quae filias Evae parturientes conturbant. praeterea si regina quaelibet vel imperatrix aut comitissa in saeculari maiestate nominis sui fastigium obtinuerit, non minus quam mulier paupercula in generatione sua fastidium anxietatis incurrit, nec alio modo onusta gemmis et auro concipit aut parit in palatio quam inops et pannosa mulier in tugurio. omnes in peccato concipiunt, omnes in dolore parturiunt, omnes Evae molestia deprimit, omnes tristitia primae matris involvit. *The Letters of Osbert of Clare, Prior of Westminster*, edited by Edward W. Williamson (London, 1929), 135-40.

[24] For detailed discussion of the medical risks associated with pregnancy see Carole Rawcliffe, 'Women, childbirth and religion in later medieval England', in *Women and Religion in Medieval England*, edited by Diana Wood (Oxford, 2003), 91-117, especially 91-95. For practical remedies available to women to counter these dangers see, for example, *The Trotula: A Medieval Compendium of Women's Medicine*, edited and translated by Monica Green (Philadelphia, 2001).

most frequently undertaken by female midwives. Citing the fourteenth-century surgeon Guy de Chauliac, Carole Rawcliffe notes that medieval obstetrics was a 'field haunted by women'.²⁵ The experiences of higher status women in particular appear to have been determined by gendered roles and expectations, with expectant women withdrawing from public society six weeks before their confinement where they were attended by matrons of suitable rank, with the only male presence likely to have been a priest.²⁶ In this context the presence of male clerics in Queen Eleanor's birthing chamber is even more striking and attests to the perceived urgency, even necessity, of the particular form of intercession specified by the King.

Divine assistance was also sought, in the form of appeals for saintly intervention or in the practices of folk medicine which often mingled Christianised practices with much older traditions.²⁷ To some extent divine interventions in childbirth conformed to similarly gendered expectations. The foremost saint of any gender associated with pregnancy and childbirth was the Virgin Mary, the antithesis to Eve whose punishment for bringing about the Fall included that she 'shalt bring forth children' in 'sorrow' (Genesis 3:16), a curse bequeathed to all womankind. The Virgin's immaculate conception and supposedly painless birth made her a potent symbol for women whose own experiences were typically so different. Mary's role as both idealised mother and intercessor of choice for mothers-to-be is attested by the growing popularity of Marian cults throughout the middle ages and the profusion of shrines, altars, images and literary depictions of her as a heavily

---

²⁵ *The Cyrurgie of Guy de Chauliac*, edited by Margaret S. Ogden, Early English Text Society, original series, 265 (London and New York, 1971), 530, cited in Rawcliffe, 'Women, childbirth and Religion', 95.

²⁶ For lying-in rituals see Becky R. Lee, 'Men's recollections of a woman's rite: medieval English men's recollections regarding the rite of purification of women after childbirth', *Gender and History*, 14 (2002), 224-41; Gail McMurray Gibson, 'Scene and obscene: seeing and performing late medieval childbirth', *Journal of Medieval and Early Modern Studies*, 29 (1999), 7-25.

²⁷ Tony Hunt, *Popular Medicine in Thirteenth-Century England* (Woodbridge, 1990); Keith Thomas, *Religion and the Decline of Magic* (London, 1984). For social and devotional practices surrounding childbirth see Elizabeth L'Estrange, *Holy Motherhood: Gender, Dynasty and Visual Culture in the Later Middle Ages* (Manchester and New York, 2008), 55-68.

pregnant or nursing mother.[28] The development of the cult of the Virgin also occasioned growing devotion to the rest of the Holy Family, particularly Mary's mother St Anne. An apocryphal figure, St Anne came to be known as a thrice-married mother of three daughters and grandmother of seven boys whose experiences were cast as a mirror of the concerns and aspirations of the women and men who constructed her saintly image.[29] A saint with a more visceral claim to the patronage of labouring women was St Margaret of Antioch, whose bursting forth unharmed from the belly of the dragon, a personification of the devil sent to torment Margaret and test her faith, was deemed analogous to the pains and perils of childbirth.[30] Features of the *vitae* of many other female saints similarly led to their association with conception, pregnancy and birth. The range of artefacts and invocations associated with the Virgin, St Anne and St Margaret alone attests to the widespread nature of belief in their efficacy amongst people of all ranks and classes and across temporal and geographical borders and the undeniable need for assistance which they were believed to fulfil.[31]

Male saints were equally capable of fulfilling the role of heavenly midwife. Child-saints such as William of Norwich (d. 1144) often displayed sympathy for other imperilled children and their mothers. Two such miracles attributed to the boy martyr recount him aiding women weakened by 'issues of blood'.[32] The physically debilitating and socially stigmatising condition suffered by the women has been identified by medical historians as the result of

[28] Miri Rubin, *Mother of God: A History of the Virgin Mary* (New Haven and London, 2009) and Jaroslav Pelikàn, *Mary Through the Centuries: Her Place in the History of Culture* (New Haven and London, 1998), 113-24.

[29] Gail McMurray Gibson, 'St Anne and the religion of childbed: some East Anglian texts and talismans', in *Interpreting Cultural Symbols: Saint Anne in Late Medieval Society*, edited by Kathleen Ashley and Pamela Sheingorn (Athens, Georgia, 1990), 95-110.

[30] Carole Hill, *Women and Religion in Late Medieval Norwich* (Woodbridge, 2010), 61-77.

[31] Hill itemises material evidence for the cults of St Anne and St Margaret of Antioch in later medieval Norwich. Hill, *Women and Religion*, 173-78. See also L'Estrange, *Holy Motherhood*, 55-68.

[32] Thomas of Monmouth, *Life and Miracles of St William of Norwich*, edited and translated by Augustus Jessopp and Montague R. James (Cambridge, 1896), 133, 169-70.

fistulae sustained during childbirth.³³ The Christological overtones of these miracles are readily apparent, casting St William in the likeness of Christ healing the woman afflicted by a perpetual issue of blood for twelve years (Mark 5: 25-34). Other male saints with less obvious connections with childbirth are likewise credited with similar miracles. Thomas Becket, for example, intervened to save both mother and child during a particularly difficult breach birth, graphically recounted by William of Canterbury (fl. 1172) in his version of the martyred archbishop's life and miracles. According to William, the parish priest who was present at the scene recalled that the only solution seemed to be to amputate the baby's trapped arm which had swollen 'equal to the thickness of a man's leg' in the hope that this would aid the delivery, but gratefully concluded that once the mother was given water to drink from Becket's shrine, 'the hand was withdrawn and the foetus turned and presented normally, all through the intervention of St Thomas'.³⁴ John Capgrave (1393-1464) recalls a similar incident in which Gilbert of Sempringham assisted a woman 'whech trauayled in byrth of a child too dayes'.³⁵

Thus Henry III's appeal to St Edmund, a male saint, is not without precedent in medieval childbed practices. However, it is notable that whilst the analogous activities of many other 'midwife' saints of both genders are found in the pages of miracle registers, this aspect of Edmund's intercessory activity is notably lacking in accounts of his life and miracles produced by the abbey at Bury. Like many saints, Edmund's miracle-working profile evolved over time to suit changing social and historical circumstances and the needs of his devotees. In the early days of his cult, for example, and in the immediate aftermath of the Norman Conquest, he is the vengeful defender of the lands and privileges of the monastic community which grew up around his remains, whereas by the fourteenth century the widespread dissemination of his cult is

---

[33] Rawcliffe, 'Women, childbirth and religion', 94.

[34] William of Canterbury, *Miraculorum Thomae Cantuariensis archiepiscopi*, in *Materials for the History of Thomas Becket*, edited by James C. Robertson, volume 1 (London, 1876), book 2, 227-28.

[35] John Capgrave, *Lives of St Augustine and St Gilbert of Sempringham*, edited by John J. Munro, Early English Text Society, original series, 140 (London, 1910), 125.

apparent and his miracles are no longer restricted to abbey lands or the nobly born: Edmund is just as likely to rescue a child from a well in rural Norfolk as he is to punish a land-hungry earl or knight.[36] This seemingly implies a stark disparity between Henry III's response to Edmund's cult and the version which was propagated by the abbey. However, I believe it is possible to discern within Edmund's *vitae* and *miraculae*, both the official and the more marginal, certain traits and tendencies which account for his invocation as miraculous midwife.

St Edmund the Virgin

One notable feature of Edmund's saintly identity which may initially seem at odds with patronage of pregnancy or childbirth is his virginity. The importance of this aspect of his saintly persona is apparent from the outset of the cult, as Edmund's first biographer, the tenth-century hagiographer Abbo of Fleury, explains the significance of the alleged incorruption of Edmund's remains:

> And how great was the holiness in this life of the holy martyr may be conjectured from the fact that his body even in death displays something of the glory of the resurrection without a trace of decay; for it must be borne in mind that they who are endued with this kind of distinction are extolled by the Catholic Fathers in the rolls of their religion as having attained the peculiar privilege of virginity, for they teach that such as have preserved their chastity till death, and have endured the stress of persecution even to the goal of martyrdom, by a just recompense are endued even here on earth, when death is past, with incorruption of the flesh ... Let us then consider what manner of man he was, who, stationed on the royal throne in the midst of worldly wealth and luxury, strove to conquer self by the incorruptibility of his flesh.[37]

---

[36] Pinner, *St Edmund, King and Martyr*, 77-101, 115-17 and 313-32.

[37] Sed de hoc sancto martyre aestimari licet, cujus sit sanctitatis in hac vita, cujus caro mortua praefert quoddam resurrectionis decus sine sui labe aliqua; quandoquidem eos, qui hujuscemodi munere donati sunt, extollant Catholici patres, suae religionis indiculo, de singulari virginitatis adepto privilegio; dicentes quod justa remuneratione etiam hic gaudent praeter mortem de carnis incorruptione, qui eam usque ad mortem servaverunt, non sine jugis martyrii valida persecutione ... Considerandum igitur quis iste fuerit, qui in regni culmine inter tot divitias et luxus saeculi semet ipsum calcata carnis petulantia vincere studuit, quod eius ostendit caro incorruptibilis. Abbo of

Abbo's *Passio* remained the definitive written version of Edmund's *vita* until the fifteenth century and is therefore the principal textual precedent by which his cult would be understood during the reign of Henry III. Abbo wrote his *Passio* for a male monastic audience in the context of the Benedictine reforms of the tenth century, of which a major tenet was the promotion of clerical celibacy.[38] In terms of its original purpose and audience it may therefore seem far removed from the practical concerns of labouring women. However, if re-imagined from the perspective of an expectant mother, Edmund, like Christ on the cross, offers a model of physical suffering which may be endured and overcome. In this respect it is significant that Abbo's depiction of Edmund is explicitly Christological; Edmund is dragged before the Viking chieftain 'like Christ before the governor Pilate', 'mocked in many ways' and 'savagely beaten' before being tied to a tree and 'tortured with terrible lashes' before being shot full of arrows and eventually beheaded.[39] The wound, which miraculously heals once Edmund's severed head is reunited with his body following the martyrdom, signifies physical regeneration and his post-mortem incorruption is therefore a signifier of his triumph over the flesh. The imagery of physical intactness and preservation of the flesh assumes alternative connotations analogous to the desire for the preservation of the woman, physically and spiritually, during and after birth; just as St Margaret burst forth from the flesh of the dragon, so too Edmund's flesh was ruptured by arrow and sword. The *exempla* offered by Edmund may be particularly compelling to an expectant mother as

---

Fleury, '*Passio Sancti Edmundi*', edited and translated by Francis Hervey in *Corolla Sancti Edmundi* (London, 1907), 6-59; XIX, 55-57. Unless stated otherwise all translations of Abbo's text will be drawn from this edition. Hervey's remains the only full modern English translation of the *Passio* although the most recent Latin scholarly edition is in *Three Lives of English Saints*, edited by Michael Winterbottom (Toronto, 1972), 67-87, from London: British Library MS Cotton Tiberius B. ii, fols 2-19v.

[38] The fullest treatment of Abbo's career and achievements is Marco Mostert, *The Political Theology of Abbo of Fleury: A Study of the Ideas about Society and Law of the Tenth-Century Monastic Reform Movement* (Hilversum, 1987), 17-18, 40-64. For the Benedictine Reforms in general see Catherine Cubitt, 'The tenth-century Benedictine Reform in England', *Early Medieval Europe*, 6.1 (1997), 77-94.

[39] Abbo, *Passio*, X; Hervey, *Corolla*, 33-35.

his wounded body corresponds to her own, whereas Margaret is more akin to the child born by the grace of divine will.

St Edmund and Fertility

Edmund's personal inviolability also extended to his kingdom. In a narrative gesture borrowed from Bede's *Ecclesiastical History*, Abbo begins his *Passio* with a description of East Anglia as a fertile but also watery and vulnerable region 'that it is washed by waters on almost every side', making it ideal terrain for the Vikings who encroach by boat along its many inlets and waterways.[40] East Anglia is therefore like the penetrable female body, associated with dampness and fluidity in medieval humoral theory, but also a fertile region which brings forth and sustains life.[41] In accordance with medieval conceptions of sacred kingship Edmund is a synecdoche of his kingdom and sacrifices his life in order to save this watery region. In death he is an even more vigorous defender of his lands and people, best exemplified in his swift and merciless despatching of the invading Danish King Sweyn Forkbeard in 1014, an event enthusiastically retold and illustrated by successive hagiographers and likely to have been depicted in the vicinity of Edmund's shrine at Bury.[42] Edmund is therefore a visible and enthusiastic defender and preserver of the integrity of his kingdom and its fertile resources.

---

[40] Abbo, *Passio*, II; Hervey, *Corolla*, 13-15.

[41] According to medieval theories of materialism all of creation was formed from the four elements of fire, air, water and earth. Regardless of sex, all four elements were believed to be present in the human body, carried by the physiological fluids or humours, but the balance of humours was believed to differ between the sexes, with men comprised mainly of the more elemental yellow bile (in which fire dominates) and blood (dominated by air), whereas women consisted principally of the more earthly elements of phlegm (mostly water) and black bile (primarily earth). For gendered understandings of humoral theory see Laura Jose, 'Monstrous conceptions: sex, madness and gender in medieval medical texts', *Comparative Critical Studies*, 5 (2008), 153-63.

[42] Pinner, *St Edmund, King and Martyr*, 228-44. See also Nicholas Rogers, 'The Frenze palimpsest', in *Tributes to Nigel J. Morgan: Context of Medieval Art: Images, Objects and Ideas*, edited by Julian Luxford and Michael A. Michael (London, 2010), 223-37.

Edmund's connection with the life and physical well-being of his kingdom is apparent from his first arrival on East Anglian soil upon his succession to the throne. In his mid-twelfth-century *De infantia Sancti Eadmundi* Geoffrey of Wells relates that the young prince knelt and gave thanks for a successful sea crossing from 'Saxony':

> At that place also, as he rose from his knees, and mounted his horse, there broke from the ground twelve springs of extraordinary clearness, which continue to flow, even in these days, to the admiration of all who behold them as they glide perpetually to the sea with a pleasant and cheerful murmur.[43]

'That place' referred to by Geoffrey is St Edmund's wells in Old Hunstanton (Norfolk), today still identified as a series of ponds in the vicinity of the church. The land responds to Edmund, acknowledging and recognising his sovereignty, and his first miracle on East Anglian soil is one associated with bringing fertility to the land via the feminine humour of life-giving water.

Similarly, Hermann relates that at the time of Edmund's translation into the newly-completed abbey church at Bury in 1089, East Anglia was in the grip of paralysing drought which threatened famine for the region. The bishop presiding over the translation ceremony ordered that the saint's body be borne outside the church and prayers offered for the ending of the long drought. Heavy rain fell and a good harvest followed.[44] Edmund's reputation as a rain-bringer and progenitor of crops persisted throughout the middle ages, as attested by Cromwell's Commissioners in 1535:

> Amongest the reliques we founde moche vanitie and superstition...divers skulls for the hedache; peces of the holie crosse able to make a hole crosse of; other reliques for rayne and certain

---

[43] '*Gaufridi de fontibus liber de infantia Sancti Eadmundi*', in *Memorials of St Edmund's Abbey*, edited by Thomas Arnold, volume 1 (London, 1890), 99-100. *De infantia* is also edited by Rodney M. Thomson, 'Geoffrey of Wells, De infantia Sancti Edmundi (BHL 2393)', *Analecta Bollandiana*, 95 (1977), 34-42. Unless stated otherwise, all citations are from Arnold's edition.

[44] Hermann, *De miraculis*, 84-85.

other superstitiouse usages, for avoiding of wedes growing in corne, with suche other.[45]

The White Bull of Bury St Edmunds

The most compelling evidence which securely locates Edmund's intercessions within the scope of human pregnancy and childbirth post-dates Henry III's appeal to the saint by more than two centuries but offers a tantalising glimpse of what may be far older practices. This is the ritual of the white bull that seems to have taken place in Bury with some regularity until at least 1533. A white bull, kept especially for the purpose in the abbey's meadow at Haberdon on the outskirts of the town, was garlanded with ribbons and flowers and processed through the streets. Women who wished to conceive would walk beside the bull, stroking its sides, until the procession reached the west gate of the monastic precinct. Here the women would leave the procession and offer prayers and votive gifts at Edmund's shrine. The importance of this ritual is attested by several fifteenth- and early sixteenth-century leases for the Haberdon meadow in which the abbey's sacrist specifies the obligation for the tenant of the meadow to keep a white bull ready and available at all times.[46] A document which seems to be from the now-lost register of sacrist John of Swaffham (c. 1471-1475), cited by antiquarian Edmund Gillingwater in the early eighteenth century, suggests that this aspect of Edmund's intercessory reputation was known outside of East Anglia:

> We made known to you by these Presents, that Father Peter Minnebode, a lay Brother of the Order of Carmelites, of the City of Gaunt [sic], on the second day of the month of June, in the year of our Lord 1474, did in the presence of many credible persons, offer at the Bier of the Glorious King, Virgin, and Martyr St Edmund, of Bury, aforesaid, one white bull, according to the ancient custom, to

---

[45] *Three Chapters of Letters Relating to the Suppression of the Monasteries*, edited by Thomas Wright, Camden Society, London, volume 26 (London, 1843), 144.

[46] London: British Library MS Harley 308, fol. 9v; William Dugdale, *Monasticon Anglicanum*, edited and translated by John Caley et al., volume 3 (London, 1846), 133; Edmund Gillingwater, *An Historical and Descriptive Account of St Edmunds Bury, in the County of Suffolk* (Bury St Edmunds, 1804), 141-49.

the honour of God, and the said glorious Martyr, in relief of the desire of a certain Noble Lady. Sealed with the Seal of our office.[47]

Cross-cultural studies attest to the ubiquity of the bull as a fundamental cultural symbol throughout millennia in the west. Jack Randolph Conrad in particular notes the enduring presence of bulls in rituals of fertility:

> Man has been fighting bulls for at least fifty thousand years ... by the dawn of recorded history man had also begun to worship them. In doing so, he wrote poetry about them, painted their portraits, moulded their images, sacrificed them, and constructed elaborate mythologies and theologies about them. More specifically, he responded strongly and fervently to the two fundamental qualities of the bull which were also the paramount masculine values: tremendous strength and great fertility. Indeed, man has always reacted more to the bull as a symbol of these two qualities than to the bull as an animal.[48]

In some western cultures, particularly southern Spain and Portugal, this association persists. In an account strikingly reminiscent of John of Swaffham's fifteenth-century description of the white bull of Bury, Gerald Brenan recalls the ritual of St Mark which is still practiced in some areas of Estremadura and Andalusia:

> A bull is caught, doped with wine until it has become gentle, and paraded through the town under the name of the saint. Women and girls caress it with Pasiphaë-like gestures, and their future fate in love and childbearing is deduced from its response to their attentions. It is commonly believed that the bull becomes gentle because the spirit of St Mark has entered into it.[49]

---

[47] Gillingwater, *Historical and Descriptive Account*, 147. See also Rodney M. Thomson, *The Archives of the Abbey of Bury St Edmunds*, Suffolk Records Society, 21 (Bury St Edmunds, 1980), 11 and 166.

[48] Jack Randolph Conrad, *The Horn and the Sword: The History of the Bull as a Symbol of Power and Fertility* (London, 1959), 9. For the history of the bull as cultural signifier see also Donald K. Sharpes, *Sacred Bull, Holy Cow: A Cultural Study of Civilisation's Most Important Animal* (New York, 2006) and Hannah Velten, *Cow* (London, 2007).

[49] Gerald Brenan, *The Face of Spain* (New York, 1951), 258-59.

Conclusion

It is possible that Henry III's appeal to Edmund to act as spiritual midwife was unique and due to his personal devotion to the saint, informed by his visits to Bury. However, reading this miracle in the context of a pre-existing and long-enduring discourse of generation and fertility renders Henry's invocation of Edmund in these circumstances more readily explicable. It also emphasises a broader methodological point as the complex interaction of saintly characteristics evident here can only be fully appreciated by considering the cult both across time and by eliding the boundaries of so-called high and low culture. It requires us to complicate the notion of 'high' and 'low' devotion as the narrative fits neatly into neither category but instead occupies a more marginal position, deriving authority, or at least inspiration, from some aspects of the official cult, but equally evincing the validity of non-hagiocentric saintly identity. Crucially, however, it relies on both perspectives to animate the source material, demonstrating the importance of an approach that incorporates multiple disciplinary perspectives. This most likely reflects something more akin to what may tentatively be assumed to be the experience of the majority of medieval devotees: at times they needed a kindly healer or a vengeful king, but sometimes they also needed protection and assistance with growing crops or in the conception and delivery of children. In reality St Edmund of East Anglia really was both 'Martir, mayde and kynge', and midwife, and more besides.

JOHN FOXE'S GOLDEN SAINTS? WAYS OF READING FOXE'S FEMALE MARTYRS IN LIGHT OF VORAGINE'S *GOLDEN LEGEND*

Fiona Kao

This chapter will look at John Foxe's (1517-1587) presentation of female martyrdom in his *Acts and Monuments*, which was first published in 1563. In the first part of this chapter I will situate Foxe's work within the context of contemporary polemic debates between Protestants and Catholics regarding beliefs in miracles and martyrdom. I will proceed to analyse extant historical scholarship addressing the presentation of Foxe's female martyrs. After which I will argue that current research fails to recognise the significance of Foxe's use of motifs, rhetoric and topoi adapted from medieval martyrologies and hagiographical works, such as Eusebius' *Ecclesiastical History* and also the *Golden Legend*. Through a close textual analysis of the accounts of three female martyrs I will demonstrate how and why, despite Foxe's strongly worded criticisms of saints' legends and miracles, he adopts and adapts hagiographical typologies, along with anecdotes that allude to miracles, in his depiction of Protestant female martyrs.

John Foxe was a fellow of Magdalen College, Oxford, where he became a member of the circle of evangelists there.[1] When Queen Mary came to the throne in 1553, he felt that he was being sought out for his Protestant faith and fled to the continent, where, in 1554, he published his *Commentarii rerum in ecclesia gestarum*, a history of the True Church (or as Foxe saw it, the Protestant Church) from John Wycliffe (d. 1384) to Reginald Peacock (*c.* 1392-*c.* 1459) and Savonarola (1452-1498). As persecution of the

---

[1] For a concise biography of John Foxe, see Thomas S. Freeman, 'John Foxe: a biography'. Accessible online: http://www.johnfoxe.org/index.php?realm=more&type=essay [accessed 10 July 2013].

Protestants intensified in England, Foxe prepared to publish a second martyrology that would incorporate contemporary Marian martyrs. The result was the Latin *Rerum in ecclesia gestarum*, printed in 1559. The *Rerum* covers the reigns of Henry VIII (1509-1547), Edward VI (1547-1553), and Mary (1553-1558).

After Mary died, Foxe returned to England, where he contemplated publishing a contemporary martyrology in English. Foxe and his patron, William Cecil, selected English as the language of the *Acts and Monuments* to ensure a broad readership. Foxe's *Acts and Monuments* was published in 1563, covering English church history from Wycliffe to the accession of Elizabeth I, though Foxe also included the earlier history of the church, a history of the papacy and expanded his writings on the Marian martyrs. Despite its size, length, and incorporation of expensive woodcuts, the *Acts and Monuments* was hugely popular and financially successful, published in no less than four editions during Foxe's lifetime and subsequently in 1570, 1576, and 1583.[2]

The text of the *Acts and Monuments* is significant not only because it records the martyrdom of approximately three hundred English Protestants who died during Mary's reign, along with their medieval predecessors, but also because it postulated a systematic attack on the Catholic Church, its assumed authority over the English Church, and its errors (according to John Foxe), such as the doctrine of transubstantiation, clerical celibacy, and auricular confession. The *Acts and Monuments* was a developing, living project which was continually adapted by John Foxe during his lifetime. As word of Foxe's tome spread, eyewitness accounts of the burnings of the martyrs, letters to and from particular martyrs, personal memoirs of the execution of the martyrs, and letters defending the honour of the 'persecutors', often written by their relatives, poured into the printshop of John Day, Foxe's publisher in London. Foxe incorporated the new material and findings from his archival research into his three subsequent editions. Foxe

---

[2] On the preparation and printing process of the *Acts and Monuments*, see Elizabeth Evenden and Thomas S. Freeman, *Religion and the Book in Early Modern England: The Making of Foxe's 'Book of Martyrs'* (Cambridge, 2011). This paper will not consider the posthumous editions of the *Acts and Monuments*.

continued to edit his work, describing and commenting on the latest political and religious events, situating these in a Protestant framework. For example, he included descriptions of the Saint Bartholomew's Day massacre (1572) and the conversion of Jews and Catholics in his 1583 edition as evidence of the impending Apocalypse. The *Acts and Monuments* is a combination of martyrology, church history, and Protestant propaganda; it is a strongly worded and sometimes overly sensational polemical tract against Catholicism and because of its popularity, it helped shape English Protestantism from the sixteenth century onward.

John Foxe presented a reformed version of church history by citing only sources that supported his claims, quoting sources out of context, rewriting his sources, and omitting sections that he did not agree with. He set at extreme opposites the 'true' Protestant Church, finding its origins in the early Christian church, and the 'false' Catholic Church that had been tainted with what he deemed to be superstitious miracles, corruption, erroneous doctrine, and abuse of power. In contrast, for Foxe, the Protestant church stemmed directly from the true teaching of Christ, the apostles, and the early church, and his Protestant martyrs were the direct descendants of the early Christian martyrs. Foxe characterised England's break from Rome as a break from her dark medieval past. Foxe presented his *Acts and Monuments* as the antithesis of medieval saints' legends and, typically, the very first events to come under fire are miracles:

> I haue oftentimes before complayned that the stories of Sayntes haue bene poudered and sawsed with diuers vntrue additions and fabulous inuentio[n]s of men, who either of a superstitious deuotion, or of a subtill practise, haue so mingle mangled their stories and liues, that almost nothing remayneth in them simple and vncorrupt.[3]

The 'stories of Sayntes' that Foxe so denigrated were most likely the *Golden Legend* and other associated works.[4] The *Golden Legend* was

---

[3] John Foxe, *Acts and Monuments* (London, 1583), 118. Available online: John Foxe, *The Unabridged Acts and Monuments Online* (HRI Online Publications, Sheffield, 2011), available from http://www.johnfoxe.org [accessed 1 January, 2011]. All citations from Foxe are from his 1583 edition unless otherwise specified.

[4] Jacobus de Voragine, *The Golden Legend*, edited by Frederick S. Ellis (Edinburgh, 1900). Accessible online: http://www.catholic-forum.com/

written around 1260 by Jacobus de Voragine, a Dominican monk, and later translated into English and published by William Caxton in 1483. The work was hugely popular in the Latin West from the thirteenth century onwards and its stories were still well known to the general public in Foxe's time. The legends typically follow a similar pattern: the saint is of noble blood, he or she stands firm in the face of persecution by his or her pagan tormentors, he or she undergoes a series of tortures and is either unharmed or miraculously healed, and eventually the saint is executed, usually by sword. For John Foxe, there were many problems with this practice of demonstrating sanctity, and miracles ranked top of the list, since saints and their miracles represented one of the errors of the Catholic Church. Foxe discarded the saints from these late medieval legendaries as suitable models for his Protestant martyrs, yet he found in the early Christian martyrs, the qualities that he so respected:

> Whose kindes of punishments although they were diuers, yet the maner of constancie in all these Martyrs was one. And yet notwithstanding the sharpenes of these so many and sundry torme[n]ts, and like cruelnes of the tormentors: yet such was the nu[m]ber of these constant Saintes that suffered, or rather such was the power of the Lord in his Saints.[5]

A major distinction that Foxe makes between the martyrs depicted in saints' legends and early Christian martyrs is that the former undergo torments without feeling pain and are divinely assisted by miracles, while the latter are patient sufferers of torments that they feel acutely. Foxe's strong distinction between the 'true' Protestant Church and the 'false' Catholic Church and between the 'superstitious' medieval saints' legends and the 'historically accurate' Protestantised martyrs' accounts has become such a dominant idea in English historiography that academics have taken Foxe's partisan view and focused primarily on the distinctions between Protestantism and Catholicism, and between pre-Reformation and post-Reformation life as a whole. It was as if the Reformation was a knife that cut English history into two clean

---

saints/golden000.htm [accessed 10 July 2013]. For a more recent edition, see *The Golden Legend: Readings on the Saints*, translated by William Granger Ryan, 2nd edn (Princeton, 2012).

[5] Foxe, *Acts and Monuments*, 57.

slices. The advent of the works of revisionist historians, such as Eamon Duffy, who argued for the existence of a continuity between pre- and post-Reformation England, has since adapted the current scholarly consensus that there indeed was a continuum between the two historical periods.[6]

This continuity becomes apparent in the diverse, and often critical, approaches to miracles and martyrdom displayed by late medieval writers, such as William Langland, Geoffrey Chaucer, and the authors of Lollard texts.[7] In the early modern period, humanists such as Desiderius Erasmus and Thomas More continued this line of invective against miracles.[8] Although devout Catholics, like More, also cautioned against miracles, it is usually the Evangelicals' polemical works that were more widely accepted in post-Reformation England, works which sharply delineated Catholicism, superstition, and miracles, on the one hand, from Protestantism, true faith, and the denunciation of miracles on the other.

These Evangelicals included William Tyndale and John Bale, who attacked miracles as a main feature in a lengthy list of Catholic errors.[9] Moreover, aside from polemical works against miracles, during the time of the Dissolution of the Monasteries, many relics

[6] Eamon Duffy, *The Stripping of the Altars: Traditional Religion in England, c. 1400-c. 1580* (New Haven and London, 1992); Martin Ingram, *Church Courts, Sex and Marriage in England, 1570-1640* (New York, 1987); Tessa Watt, *Cheap Print and Popular Piety, 1550-1640* (New York and Cambridge, 1991); Ronald Hutton, *The Rise and Fall of Merry England: The Ritual Year 1400-1700* (Oxford and New York, 1994); Alexandra Walsham, *Providence in Early Modern England* (Oxford and New York, 1999) and Alexandra Walsham, *The Reformation of the Landscape: Religion, Identity, and Memory in Early Modern Britain and Ireland* (New York, 2011).

[7] William Langland's *Piers Plowman* (ca. 1360-1387); Geoffrey Chaucer's *Canterbury Tales* (1475); *The Works of a Lollard Preacher: The Sermon 'Omni plantacio', the Tract 'Fundamentum aliud nemo potest ponere' and the Tract 'De oblacione iugis sacrificii'*, edited by Anne Hudson, Early English Text Society, original series, 317 (New York, 2001).

[8] Desiderius Erasmus, 'The Shipwreck', 'The Apparition', and 'The Religious Pilgrimage', in *The Whole Familiar Colloquies of Desiderius Erasmus of Rotterdam*, translated by Nathan Bailey (London, 1877); Thomas More, *The dialogue concerning heresies*, Book 1, Chapters 14-15, in *The Complete Works of St Thomas More*, edited by Thomas M. C. Lawler et al., 15 vols (New Haven and London, 1981).

[9] William Tyndale, *The Obedience of a Christian Man* (Antwerp, 1528). John Bale, *The Actes of English Votaryes* (Antwerp, 1546).

were exposed as forgeries. For example, the Rood of Grace on which a figure was supposed to miraculously move and speak was exposed to be moved by levers and wires; the Holy Blood at Hailes Abbey was discovered to be that of a duck. Protestant authors acknowledged that miracles occurred in biblical times but they argued that these miraculous deeds had become extinct and that Catholic miracles were either fraudulent or were 'lying wonders' performed by Satan and false prophets, which Christ had forewarned would proliferate in the Last Days. However, as Alexandra Walsham has pointed out, despite the Protestant claim that miracles no longer existed, they were unwilling to completely relinquish the functions of miracles, thus 'in the guise of providence [the Protestants] were conveniently able to reclaim essentially the same kind of divine approbation'.[10]

Many Catholic authors, on the other hand, assumed a different approach to miracles. While earlier scholars argued that reformed Catholicism distanced itself from miracles, similar to Protestantism,[11] recent scholarship has offered more nuanced interpretations of the continuity and changes in attitudes towards miracles both before and after the Reformation.[12] In 1563 the

[10] Alexandra Walsham, 'Miracles in Post-Reformation England', in *Signs, Wonders, Miracles: Representations of Divine Power in the Life of the Church*, edited by Kate Cooper and Jeremy Gregory, Studies in Church History, 41 (Woodbridge, 2005), 287.

[11] Jean Delumeau, *Catholicism between Luther and Voltaire* (London, 1977); John Bossy, 'The Counter Reformation and the people of Catholic Europe', *Past and Present*, 47 (1970), 51-70; John Bossy, *Christianity in the West, 1400-1700* (Oxford, 1985); and Robert Muchembled, *Popular Culture and Elite Culture in France, 1400-1750*, translated by Lydia Cochrane (Baton Rouge and London, 1985).

[12] Louis Chatellier, *The Europe of the Devout: The Catholic Reformation and the Formation of a New Society* (Cambridge, 1989); David Gentilcore, *From Bishop to Witch: The System of the Sacred in Early Modern Terra d'Otranto* (Manchester, 1992); Duffy, *The Stripping of the Altars*; Philip Soergel, *Wondrous in his Saints: Counter-Reformation Propaganda in Bavaria* (Berkeley, 1993); Louis Chatellier, *The Religion of the Poor: Rural Missions in Europe and the Formation of Modern Catholicism, c. 1500-c. 1800* (Cambridge, 1997); R. Po-Chia Hsia, *The World of Catholic Renewal, 1540-1770* (Cambridge, 1998); Michael Mullett, *The Catholic Reformation* (London and New York, 1999); and Robert Bireley, *The Refashioning of Catholicism, 1450-1700: A Reassessment of the Counter Reformation* (Basingstoke, 1999); Walsham, *Providence in Early Modern England*; Alexandra Walsham, 'Miracles and the Counter-Reformation Mission to England', *The Historical Journal*, 46.4

Council of Trent ordered the eradication of all superstition associated with pilgrimages, images, and relics but reaffirmed the veneration of saints, their relics and their representation. The Catholic Church did not reject the notion that objects could elicit miracles, but sought instead to bring these objects under clerical control. By presenting miracles as Providence, Protestant writers did not completely reject the existence of miracles in their contemporary world. Similarly, many Catholic authors continued to incorporate miracles into newly written hagiographies of contemporary Catholic saints. These writers contested the Protestant claim that miracles no longer existed, claiming that miracles continued to prove God's favour to the Catholic Church.

Yet, despite the vast array of scholarship written on this topic, there has been little research conducted into the use of medieval hagiographical literature and conventions in Protestant texts, including John Foxe's *Acts and Monuments*. Before I delve into Foxe's adaptation of the virgin martyr hagiographical trope, I will first give an overview of the contended issues concerning female martyrdom both in early modern polemics and recent scholarly debate.

In his presentation of female martyrs John Foxe faced a dilemma. He wanted his readers to view his martyrs as examples not only of Christian constancy but also of virtuous female behaviour. On the one hand, his female martyrs needed to inveigh against Catholic authority and appear as Christ's soldiers for the Protestant truth; on the other hand, they had to conform to the social constraints placed on women in sixteenth-century England, and be considered modest, pious, and morally impeccable. Foxe's presentation of his female martyrs attracted much attention from contemporary critics, including Thomas Harding and Robert Persons, who denounced these martyred women for their audacity, disobedience, and outspokenness. One of the strategies that Foxe adopted to reconcile the concepts of womanhood and martyrdom

(2003), 779-815; Marc Forster, *Catholic Germany from the Reformation to the Enlightenment* (Basingstoke, 2007); Trevor Johnson, *Magistrates, Madonnas and Miracles: The Counter Reformation in the Upper Palatinate* (Farnham, 2009); and Philip Soergel, *Miracles and the Protestant Imagination: The Evangelical Wonder Book in Reformation Germany* (New York, 2012).

was to model his contemporary female martyrs on pre-existing tropes, including that of the virgin martyr exhibited in saints' legends.

Several scholars have noted the difficulties Foxe experienced when attempting to reconcile conflicting concepts of womanhood and martyrdom. Carole Levin points out that '[t]hough Foxe is certainly concerned with Christian virtues for women, in certain ways the examples in *The Book of Martyrs* not only reinforce, but also modify this point of view'.[13] Levin investigates five female martyrs in the *Acts and Monuments*, each exhibiting varying levels of female conformity. She categorises Foxe's women into three groups: those who succeeded in manipulating men, those who did not succeed, and the 'wild cards' which fit into neither of the two previous categories. Levin flags up the problems of 'too neatly categorising the way Foxe presents women'.[14] Yet, there is no further investigation into how Foxe alleviates the tension between the women's behaviour and contemporary womanly ideals. In a similar strain, Steven Mullaney seeks the reason behind why Foxe chose to mould certain women into models of female virtue and not others. He states that Foxe attributes the courage of his female martyrs to God and simply concludes that 'such women do not violate the period's insistence ... that women be chaste, silent, and obedient'.[15] Instead they are 'resolved in their deaths but neither remonstrative nor overly demonstrative, less individual agents of resistance than vessels taken over by "the Lord Omnipotent" who has chosen to possess them'.[16] In other words, Mullaney states that since Foxe's women were possessed by God, their disorderly behaviour could be thus excused.

Furthermore, Susan Wabuda looks at *The Letters of the Martyrs*, a collection of letters written by several Protestant martyrs recorded

---

[13] Carole Levin, 'Women in *The Book of Martyrs* as models of behavior in Tudor England', *International Journal of Women's Studies*, 4 (1981), 196.

[14] Levin, 'Women in *The Book of Martyrs*', 205.

[15] Steven Mullaney, 'Reforming resistance: class, gender, and legitimacy in Foxe's *Book of Martyrs*', in *Print, Manuscript and Performance: The Changing Relations of the Media in Early Modern England*, edited by Arthur F. Marotti and Michael D. Bristol (Columbus, 2000), 243.

[16] Mullaney, 'Reforming resistance', 243.

in Foxe's writings.[17] Wabuda analyses how the editor of the collection of letters, Henry Bull, suppressed the contribution of women in these letters since he was very concerned about their active participation in theological discussions.[18] Similarly, Thomas Freeman has discovered that Foxe tried to conceal the theological contributions of the female supporters of his male martyrs.[19] Freeman remarks that 'Foxe was careful to force [his female martyrs] into a procrustean paradigm, modeled on that employed by Eusebius to describe female martyrs in the early church, of the Holy Spirit working through weaker instruments to confound the mighty'.[20] Susanna Monta picks up Mullaney's strength-within-weakness theme and Freeman's Eusebian allusion, noting that Foxe 'attempts to present gender transgression as testimonial validation while also containing the more radical implications of such a project'.[21] Just as Mullaney argues that the female martyrs' 'strength is not their own' but 'visited as it is upon them by God', Monta claims that 'the rhetoric of strength-within-weakness serves a powerful testimonial function, while that testimonial purpose legitimates defiant speech'.[22]

Besides the 'strength-within-weakness' strategy proposed by Mullaney, Monta, and Freeman, Megan Hickerson has proposed another strategy. She states that Foxe's female martyrs were:

> Types not of virtuous mortal womanhood, or even of godly Elizabethan Protestantism, but of the true persecuted church herself ...

---

[17] 'Certain most godly, fruitful and comfortable letters of such true Saintes and holy Martyrs as in the late bloodye persecution gaue their lyues' [RSTC 5886], edited by Henry Bull and attributed to Miles Coverdale (London, 1564).

[18] Susan Wabuda, 'Henry Bull, Miles Coverdale, and the making of Foxe's *Book of Martyrs*', in *Martyrs and Martyrologies*, Studies in Church History, 30 (Oxford, 1993), 245-48.

[19] Thomas S. Freeman, '"The Good Ministrye of Godlye and Vertuouse Women": the Elizabethan martyrologists and the female supporters of the Marian martyrs', *The Journal of British Studies*, 39 (2000), 26.

[20] Freeman, 'The Good Ministrye', 26.

[21] Susanna Brietz Monta, 'Foxe's female martyrs and the sanctity of transgression', *Renaissance and Reformation*, 25 (2001), 4.

[22] Mullaney, 'Reforming resistance', 243. Monta, 'Sanctity of transgression', 7.

Foxe's disorderly women martyrs thus serve not as models for virtuous female behaviour, but as models for disobedience.[23]

Hickerson argues that Foxe made use of earlier reformers' revisions of the Bride of Christ trope, which no longer represented the physical purity of virginity but rather a spiritual purity. According to Hickerson, Foxe contrasted the spirituality of the Protestant Church as the Bride of Christ with the carnality of the Catholic Church as the Whore of Babylon.

These approaches to Foxe's presentation of female martyrs are not without their limitations. Firstly, Foxe directly alludes to the Bride of Christ paradigm only three times in his description of the Marian female martyrs (namely for Joan Lashford, Elizabeth Folkes, and Mrs Prest).[24] It is difficult to argue then, that this was one of Foxe's main strategies to reconcile womanhood and martyrdom when it was so scarcely applied. Secondly, Foxe does not adopt the strength-within-weakness paradigm as extensively as scholars claim.[25] In several descriptions of female defiance, Foxe does not use the paradigm to temper the women's defiant behaviour, but instead allows these women to freely criticise Catholicism. Moreover, though this paradigm has been attributed to the early Christian martyrs, especially to Eusebius, Eusebius did not actually use the strength-within-weakness paradigm specifically for women.[26] In fact, for Eusebius, the 'weakness' in the 'strength-

---

[23] Megan Hickerson, *Making Women Martyrs in Tudor England* (Houndmills, Basingstoke, 2005), 161.

[24] Foxe, *Acts and Monuments*, 1882, 2032 and 2074.

[25] For examples, see Foxe, *Acts and Monuments*, 1882, 1917, 1935, 2004, 2043, 2073. In the case of Elizabeth Cooper, we see the opposite of the strength-in-weakness paradigm. She 'a little shronke thereat, with a voyce crying once, ha' and Simon Miller 'willed her to bee strong'. See Foxe, *Acts and Monuments*, 2029.

[26] For works that deal with the link between Eusebius and Foxe, see Thomas S. Freeman, '"Great searching out of bookes and autors": John Foxe as an Ecclesiastical Historian', unpublished doctoral thesis (Rutgers University, 1995); Gretchen E. Minton, '"The Same Cause and like Quarell": Eusebius, John Foxe, and the evolution of ecclesiastical history', *Church History*, 71 (2002), 715-42; Robert A. Markus, 'Church history and early church historians', in *The Materials, Sources and Methods of Ecclesiastical History*, edited by Derek Baker, Studies in Church History, 11 (Oxford, 1975). Elizabeth Clark, 'Eusebius on women in early church history', in *Eusebius,*

within-weakness' was human weakness, not specifically female weakness.[27] Thirdly, Freeman notes that Foxe's suppression of the theological contribution of the female supporters of male martyrs stems from the lack of preexisting models for 'women who did not die for the gospel'.[28] In other words, if a woman eventually died a martyr's death, her problematic, unwomanly behaviour could be excused since she had a martyr's privileges. However, when we examine the *Acts and Monuments*, Foxe's decision on whether a woman could behave in a disorderly manner or make theological contributions does not directly correlate with whether she eventually died a martyr's death. Freeman's assertion that 'it was one thing for godly women to instruct or upbraid agents of the Antichrist, and quite another for them to be lecturing, advising, or arguing theological matters with godly men' does ring true.[29] Whether Foxe interfered in the presentation of his female martyrs did not depend on whether the women eventually died a martyr's death, but on whom these women were attacking.

Finally, the main limitation of current scholarship about both Foxe's presentation of female martyrdom and his conception of martyrdom in general is that Protestant martyrology is still considered to be unrelated to medieval hagiography, even in the light of recent historical interpretations which emphasise the continuum between pre-Reformation and post-Reformation England. Medieval hagiography is presented as nothing more than a 'dark superstition' to be contrasted with Foxe's writings. This emphasis fails to recognise the significance of Foxe's incorporation of motifs, topoi, and rhetoric from Eusebius' *Ecclesiastical History* and also from medieval hagiographical collections, including the *Golden Legend*, in his presentation of contemporary Protestant female martyrs.

Christianity, and Judaism, edited by Harold W. Attridge and Gohei Hata (Detroit, 1992), 256-69, at 259.

[27] Eusebius utilised the strength-within-weakness trope both for the female martyr Blandina and the male martyr Germanicus. Eusebius, *The Ecclesiastical History*, translated by Kirsopp Lake, volume 1 (Cambridge, Massachusetts, 1926), 415, 427 and 343.

[28] Freeman, 'Good Ministrye', 27.

[29] Freeman, 'Good Ministrye', 27.

In the remainder of this chapter I will argue that, despite Foxe's constant protestations distancing his martyrology from what he considers to be the 'superstitious, fabulous, and false' medieval legends, despite his assertions that his martyrology is the successor of 'true' and 'historically accurate' martyrologies such as that of Eusebius, Foxe still makes use of models found in both Eusebius' *Ecclesiastical History* and the *Golden Legend* to demonstrate that his martyred men and women are the heirs of the early Christian martyrs. In order to demonstrate this, I will present a close textual analysis of three of Foxe's accounts of female martyrdom: those of Rose Allin, Joyce Lewis and Mrs Prest.

'I shall not swimme in that See': Rose Allin and Divine Analgesia

The woodcut 'The burning of Rose Allins hande, by Edmund Tyrrell, as she was going to fetch drinke for her Mother, lying sicke in bedde' is one of the main woodcut images of female martyrdom in the *Acts and Monuments*.[30] In this specific example, three scenes of the past, present, and future are conflated. To the left is the pictorial narration of Rose Allin's father, William Mount, praying at the bedside of his sick wife, Alice Mount. Alice reclines in bed, covered up to her arms in her blanket, her head tilted as she listens to the approaching footsteps of men surrounding her house at two in the morning. The central part of the woodcut is given to the showdown between Edmund Tyrrell and Rose Allin, while three men look on in the background. Behind Rose Allin is a painting depicting the family's burning at the stake, as the sun penetrates the thick clouds and shines upon the holy family like a heavenly spotlight.[31]

The account of Rose Allin is one of the most dramatic and shocking narrations of female martyrdom in the *Acts and Monuments*. According to John Foxe, the Mount family 'refrayned themselues from the vnsauery seruice of the Popish Churche, and

---

[30] Foxe, *Acts and Monuments*, 2030.

[31] The picture in the woodcut is too small to decipher whether there are three or four people at the stake. The Mount family was burned in a group of four with John Johnson in the castle yard of Colchester on the afternoon of 2 August 1557.

freque[n]ted the company of good men and women which gaue themselues diligently to reading, inuocating, and calling vpon the name of God through Christ'.[32] This behaviour aroused the suspicion of the priest Sir Thomas Tye who reported their behaviour to the Catholic authorities, Lord Darcy and eventually Bishop Bonner. Subsequently, Edmund Tyrrell and his men arrested the Mounts at their house. Foxe's detailed account described an anecdote that occurred during the arrest: Alice Mount asked her daughter, Rose Allin, to fetch some water for her, for she was 'very ill at ease'.[33] As Rose Allin returned with the pitcher of water in her hand, 'Tyrrel met her, & willed to geue her father & mother good cou[n]sell, and to aduertise them to be better Catholicke people'.[34] She replied that her parents had the Holy Ghost as their instructor. Tyrrell exclaimed that she would not be able to suffer the pain of burning.

What started out as a conversation between Tyrrell and the water-fetching daughter quickly evolved into a dramatic confrontation between a male torturer and a young woman. Tyrrell asked his associates, 'Syrs thys gossip wil burne: do ye not thinke it?' To which one of the men replied, 'proue her, and you shall see what she will do by and by'.[35] Their possible expectations that she could not withstand the pain of burning were proved false. Foxe describes in detail the gruesome scene that ensued: 'Then that cruell Tyrrill taking the candell from her, held her wrest, and the burning candell vnder her hande, burning crosse wise ouer the backe thereof, so long till the very sinowes crackt a su[n]der'.[36] When Rose Allin did not react in the way Tyrrell had hoped, Tyrrell exploded with fury as he roared, 'ha strong whore, thou shamelesse beast, thou beastly whore. &c'.[37]

---

[32] Foxe, *Acts and Monuments*, 2030.
[33] Foxe, *Acts and Monuments*, 2030.
[34] Foxe, *Acts and Monuments*, 2030.
[35] Foxe, *Acts and Monuments*, 2030.
[36] Foxe, *Acts and Monuments*, 2031.
[37] Foxe, *Acts and Monuments*, 2031.

The theme of the furious torturer and the serenely calm martyr can be traced back to Jewish 'martyrologies'.[38] The distinction between the tyrant's rage and the martyrs' sublimity features prominently in 4 Maccabees, which was written in either the first century BCE or first century CE, and features the martyrdom of a mother and her seven sons. After the martyrs had spoken, 'the tyrant was not only exasperated against them as being refractory, but enraged with them as being ungrateful'.[39] The author continues to describe how 'by means of the reasoning which is praised by God, [the martyrs] mastered their passions'.[40] The mother is used as a particularly edifying example. The author praises her: 'O holy mother of a nation avenger of the law, and defender of religion, and prime bearer in the battle of the affections! O thou nobler in endurance than males, and more manly than men in patience!'.[41] This contrast between rage, on the one hand, and a controlled emotional response, on the other, is influenced by the classical philosophy that reason should rule over the passions. The martyrs demonstrate that they are superior to the persecutor; even the mother, a woman, is manlier than the tyrant.[42]

This contrast between the raging persecutor and the unperturbed martyr is similarly praised in early Christian

---

[38] There is as yet no scholarly consensus on whether the concept of martyrdom originated in Christian texts or whether earlier or contemporary Jewish texts can be said to be 'martyrological works'. See William H. C. Frend, *Martyrdom and Persecution in the Early Church: A Study of a Conflict from the Maccabees to Donatus* (Oxford, 1965); William Horbury, 'The Jewish Dimension', in *Early Christianity: Origins and Evolution to AD 600: In Honour of W.H.C. Frend*, edited by Ian Hazlett (Nashville, Tennessee, 1991); Arthur J. Droge and James D. Tabor, *A Noble Death: Suicide and Martyrdom among Christians and Jews in Antiquity* (New York, 1992). Glen W. Bowersock, *Martyrdom and Rome* (Cambridge, New York, and Melbourne, 1995); Daniel Boyarin, *Dying for God: Martyrdom and the Making of Christianity and Judaism* (Stanford, 1999); Shmuel Shepkaru, *Jewish Martyrs in the Pagan and Christian Worlds* (New York, 2008) and Timothy Barnes, *Early Christian Hagiography and Roman History* (Tübingen, 2010).

[39] 4 Maccabees, 9:10.

[40] 4 Maccabees, 13:3.

[41] 4 Maccabees, 15:29.

[42] Stephen D. Moore and Janice Capel Anderson, '"Taking it Like a Man": masculinity in 4 Maccabees', *Journal of Biblical Literature*, 117.2 (1998), 255.

martyrologies. In Eusebius' depiction of Blandina's suffering in the arena, her torturers exhibit their exasperation:

> Filled with such power that she was released and rescued from those who took turns in torturing her in every way from morning until evening, and they themselves confessed that they were beaten, for they had nothing left to do to her, and they marveled that she still remained alive, seeing that her whole body was broken and opened, and they testified that any one of these tortures was sufficient to destroy life, even when they had not been magnified and multiplied.[43]

Moreover, Eusebius emphasises the extreme torments that the martyrs experienced and their heroic endurance. Eusebius describes how, in the case of Apollonia, the Romans 'pil[ed] up a pyre before the city' and 'threatened to burn her alive, if she refused to recite along with them their blasphemous sayings'. She 'asked for a brief space, and, being released, without flinching she leaped into the fire and was consumed'.[44] The readers get the sense that Apollonia felt the pain but 'without flinching' faced it courageously. In the account of Potamiaena, the judge, Aquila, 'after inflicting severe tortures upon her entire body, at last threatened to hand her over to the gladiators for bodily insult, and that, when after a brief period of reflection she was asked what her decision was, she made a reply which involved from their point of view something profane'.[45] Eusebius does not tell us what exactly she said but directs his readers' attention to her suffering: 'she right nobly endured the end, boiling pitch being poured slowly and little by little over different parts of her body from head to toe. Such was the contest waged by this maiden celebrated in song'.[46] In Blandina's case, as her persecutors inflicted more and more creative forms of torture, all she said was 'I am a Christian woman and nothing wicked happens among us'.[47] In another round of public torturing in the arena, Eusebius focuses on the sufferings that Blandina underwent but does not relate anything that she said except that she 'encouraged Ponticus, the boy [and her fellow martyr], until he

[43] Eusebius, *Ecclesiastical History*, 5.1, volume 1, 415.
[44] Eusebius, *Ecclesiastical History*, 6.41, volume 2, 103.
[45] Eusebius, *Ecclesiastical History*, 6.5, volume 2, 25-27.
[46] Eusebius, *Ecclesiastical History*, 6.5, volume 2, 25-27.
[47] Eusebius, *Ecclesiastical History*, 5.1, volume 1, 415.

gave up his spirit'.⁴⁸ One obvious but nonetheless important point to make is that forbearance is by no means limited to female martyrs but can be found among male martyrs as well.

While Eusebius' martyrs suffered various creative methods of punishment patiently, the saints depicted in the *Golden Legend* were not as even-tempered and taciturn. In St Lucy's legend, Paschasius, the judge, threatens to take Lucy to a brothel, yet neither one thousand men nor one thousand yoke of oxen could budge her. The judge then had a roaring fire built around her, boiling oil poured on her, and urine drenched on her to chase away magic – all to no avail. Voragine records that 'at this point the consul's friends, seeing how distressed he was, plunged a dagger into the martyr's throat', but Lucy still did not die, indeed she was even able to make a lengthy speech.⁴⁹ St Agnes, again depicted in the *Golden Legend*, made similar scathing remarks: when the prefect's son asked her to marry him, she replied, 'go away, you spark that lights the fire of sin, you fuel of wickedness, you food of death! I am already pledged to another lover!'.⁵⁰ The prefect, knowing of his son's lovesickness, tried to win Agnes over with sweet words but she 'met this mixture of cajolery and menace with derision'.⁵¹

Similarly, St Anastasia's actions, who featured in the *North English Legendary*, produced during the fourteenth century, brought about much humiliation to her persecutor. The pagan prince who desired Anastasia's beautiful handmaidens locked the maids up in a storeroom formerly used for kitchen utensils. One day, he went into the room to satisfy his lust with them, but thinking the pots and ladles were the maids, he 'satisfied his wicked desires' with the crockery.⁵² Sometimes the female saint did more than just hurt a judge's pride; she could become physically violent and injure her torturer. In William Paris' legend of St Christine, the judge cut out Christine's tongue but she threw the piece of

---

⁴⁸ Eusebius, *Ecclesiastical History*, 5.1, volume 1, 433.
⁴⁹ Jacobus de Voragine, *The Golden Legend: Readings on the Saints*, translated by William Granger Ryan, volume 1 (Princeton, 1993), 27-29.
⁵⁰ Voragine, *Golden Legend*, volume 1, 102.
⁵¹ Voragine, *Golden Legend*, volume 1, 102.
⁵² Winstead, *Chaste Passions*, 45-48.

tongue at him and blinded his eye.[53] At other times, the female saint caused financial damage. St Barbara, in the *South English Legendary*, cursed the shepherd who had betrayed her secret to her father and turned the shepherd's sheep into flies.[54]

From the above examples, we can see that the presentation of female martyrs in Jewish and early Christian martyrologies and in hagiographical collections provide certain motifs which later authors could draw on. The martyrologies provide a contrast between the calm patience of the martyr and the furious rage of the persecutors, while in the later medieval legends, both sides seem to be just as furious at each other. The difference is that, in the latter, the persecutors are outraged by their own shame, while the female saints are physical vessels of divine wrath.[55] Secondly, the female martyrs in early Christian martyrologies appear taciturn, while those in the *Golden Legend* tend to be eloquent or even verbally or physically abusive. Thirdly, while the saints in the *Golden Legend* never feel pain and do not need to 'endure' anything let alone suffer anything patiently, the female martyrs in Eusebius are noted for their heroic forbearance.

Returning to Rose Allin, the deliberate contrast between the furious Tyrrell and the unflappable Rose Allin follows the typological presentation of the calm martyr and the furious torturer featured in the writings of Eusebius.[56] However, as further details of Rose Allin's heroic forbearance are revealed, Foxe's allusions echo more closely those of Voragine rather than Eusebius. When Rose Allin was in prison, she told a fellow prisoner about 'this cruell act of the sayd Tirrell' and stated, 'while my one hand ... was a burning, I hauing a pot in my other hand, might haue laid him on [th]e face with it, if I had would? for no ma[n] held my hand to let me therin'.[57] This possibility of retaliation is quite a shocking

[53] Winstead, *Chaste Passions*, 68.
[54] Winstead, *Chaste Passions*, 42.
[55] On divine wrath and charitable hatred, see Alexandra Walsham, *Charitable Hatred: Tolerance and Intolerance in England, 1500-1700* (Manchester and New York, 2006).
[56] Foxe compares Rose Allin's hand-burning to the burning of the hand of Gaius Mucius Scaevola, a Roman soldier, in Livy's *History of Rome*. See Foxe, *Acts and Monuments*, 2031.
[57] Foxe, *Acts and Monuments*, 2031.

statement in itself, and it is worth noting that none of Eusebius' female martyrs ever threatened to physically injure her persecutor. Indeed both male and female martyrs were characterised by their patient suffering. The closest we get to the possibility of a female martyr wishing harm upon her persecutor is Potamiaena, who told the judge something 'profane'.

Rose Allin was asked by the prisoner as to how she could endure the pain of having her hand burned. She replied, '[A]t first it was some griefe to her, but afterward, the longer she burned, the lesse she felt, or well neare none at all'.[58] Foxe was ambiguous about whether Rose Allin did not feel the pain because of her forbearance or whether she was divinely assisted. This is an allusion to perhaps one of the most typically hagiographical elements in saints' legends – divine analgesia. Many of the saints depicted in the *Golden Legend* performed miracles when they were tortured – either their torturers were struck down by divine vengeance or the saints were healed immediately. Furthermore, these martyred saints did not appear to feel the pain of their torture. For example, in St Lucy's legend, despite having been burned alive, scalded with boiling oil and stabbed in the throat, she was still able to declare that she had become the protectress of the city of Syracusa.[59]

Foxe's ambiguous attitude toward the miracle of divine analgesia can be found not only in Rose Allin's story but also in his reworkings of hagiographical material. Though Foxe claimed that his sources were the works of more respectable authors such as Prudentius, Bergomensis, Basil the Great, Antoninus, and Ado, and not 'superstitious' works like the *Golden Legend*, his *Acts and Monuments* is not completely excised of miraculous elements. Foxe tampered with some forms of miracles by either removing them completely or reporting them and then dismissing them with a caveat that the readers should use their own judgment. However, there were some types of miracles that Foxe was more ambiguous about and divine analgesia was one of them. For example, though Foxe states directly that he omitted St Katherine's spiritual marriage to Christ and her debate with the fifty philosophers, he is

---

[58] Foxe, *Acts and Monuments*, 2031.
[59] Voragine, *Golden Legend*, volume 1, 29.

ambiguous about whether St Katherine felt the pain of her torture, claiming simply that: 'after she proued the racke, and the foure sharpe cutting wheeles, hauing at last her head cut off with the sword, so she finished her martyrdome'.[60] Though Foxe cautions his readers about the miraculous way in which St Eugenia was saved from each of her tortures, stating that; 'all which Legendary miracles I leaue to the Reader to iudge of them, as shal seeme good vnto him', we are left unsure as to whether Eugenia felt the pain of all these tortures and whether Foxe's caution applies to the miracle of divine analgesia.[61] Foxe's attitude towards St Cecilia's tortures is also revealing. St Cecilia survived a boiling bath and continued to live for three days after four strokes were struck at her neck. Foxe comments that these, along with how an angel was the keeper of her virginity, are 'straunge miracles', and concludes:

> But as touchinge these miracles, as I doo not dispute whether they be true or fabulous: so bycause they haue no grou[n]d vpon any auncient or graue authors, but taken out of certayne newe ledgends, I do therefore refer them thether from whence they came.[62]

Nevertheless, there are also instances in which it is more obvious that the saints depicted by John Foxe did feel pain, though these are not changes made by Foxe but descriptions already found in his source texts. For example, Foxe's legend of St Agnes ends with, 'The executioner then with his bloudy hand ... at one stroke cutteth off her head, & by such short & swift death doth he preuente her of [the] payne therof',[63] which clearly echoes Foxe's cited source, Prudentius: 'Thus was her ardent longing fulfilled at last/ For with one blow the soldier struck off her head/ And speedy death prevented all sense of pain'.[64] In Eulalia's legend, which Foxe also cites from Prudentius, Foxe describes the tortures Eulalia underwent until she, 'desiring swift death, opened her mouth and

---

[60] Foxe, *Acts and Monuments*, 118.
[61] Foxe, *Acts and Monuments*, 97.
[62] Foxe, *Acts and Monuments*, 98.
[63] Foxe, *Acts and Monuments*, 118.
[64] Prudentius, 'The Passion of Agnes', in *The Poems of Prudentius*, translated by Sister M. Clement Eagan (first published 1962, Washington D.C., 1981), 278.

swalowed the flame, and so rested shee in peace'.⁶⁵ Prudentius similarly describes this incident:

> Fed by her hair, the enveloping flames
>
> Mount to her face, and surrounding her head,
>
> Blaze up above it in vehement rage.
>
> Thirsting for heaven, the virgin elect
>
> Drinks in the fire with impetuous lips.⁶⁶

Based on the examples above, we can conclude that Foxe was ambiguous about the miracle of divine analgesia. If his original source portrays a saint who felt pain, he would retain this description, though if his source material depicts a saint protected by divine analgesia, albeit of potentially miraculous origins, he reproduced this description. Divine analgesia was not among the fraudulent miracles that Foxe attacked the Catholic Church for and may have been replicated as a feature within his Protestant martyrological depiction of Rose Allin.

If Foxe had not provided details of Rose Allin's later conversation, her behaviour would have fit into the general mould expected of a Eusebian-style martyr. In this suspended moment of possible brain-bashing violence, Foxe alludes to the plethora of violent female saints in the *Golden Legend*. Yet, Rose Allin continued and said, 'But I thanke God ... with all my hart, I did it not'.⁶⁷ The reader is unsure whether he or she should let out a sigh of relief or disappointment as Foxe continues to describe Rose Allin's examination:

> Rose Allyn ... being examined of auricular confession, goyng to the church to heare Masse, of the Popish seuen sacramentes &c. aunswered stoutlye that they stanke in the face of God ... for they were the members of Antichriste, and so shuld haue (if they repented not) the reward of Antichrist. Being asked further, what she could saye of the Sea of the Bishop of Rome ... she aunswered boldly ... As for hys

---

⁶⁵ Foxe, *Acts and Monuments*, 117.

⁶⁶ Prudentius, 'Hymn in honor of the Passion of the Most Holy Martyr Eulalia', in *The Poems of Prudentius*, 135.

⁶⁷ Foxe, *Acts and Monuments*, 2031.

> See ... it is for Crowes, kytes, owles and Rauens to swimme in, such as you be, for by [the] grace of God I shall not swimme in that See.

Again, Rose Allin's lengthy and stinging reply resembles the retorts found in the *Golden Legend* far more closely than the reticence of the martyrs presented by Eusebius. However, when we come to Rose Allin's death, we find a typically Eusebian martyr: when Allin and her fellow martyrs were brought to their execution site, the martyrs 'were ioyfully tyed to the stakes, calling vpon the name of God, and exhorting the people earnestly to flee from Idolatry' and 'suffered their martyrdome with ... triumphe and ioye'.[68]

When we compare Foxe's presentation of Rose Allin with the martyrs of Eusebius and those of the *Golden Legend*, we can draw several conclusions. First, concerning the contrast between the raging persecutor and the calm martyr, Rose Allin underwent the burning of her hand patiently as one would expect a Eusebian-style martyr to behave. Second, while Eusebius' female martyrs were usually either silent or taciturn, the female martyrs in the *Golden Legend* were frequently outspoken and prone to feisty bouts of verbal sparring. The rhetoric that Rose Allin used and her insolent attitude towards her persecutors are so reminiscent of the invectives in the *Golden Legend*, that if Foxe had not included the examination topics, namely, auricular confession and papal authority, the reader might think he or she is reading the legend of Saint Rose Allin![69] Thirdly, concerning whether Rose Allin felt pain, her description of how she at first felt pain but then did not feel pain anymore falls ambiguously between Eusebian forbearance and the divine analgesia of the *Golden Legend*. The martyrdom of Rose Allin is a crafty blend of both Eusebian and Voragian elements.

Foxe adopted medieval hagiographical conventions in the story of Rose Allin in order to access its polemical power along with that

---

[68] Foxe, *Acts and Monuments*, 2033.
[69] As Winstead has pointed out, late medieval hagiography gives the best examples of such invectives. The disorderly behaviour of virgin martyrs is subsumed in lavish prayers and long passages of devotion in early medieval hagiography while late 'literary' medieval hagiography including the works of Capgrave, Bokenham, and Lydgate rewrite their virgin martyrs into decorous gentlewomen. See Winstead, *Virgin Martyrs*.

of the early Christian martyrological style. What Foxe was most concerned about in his depiction of martyrs was one theme – that these martyrs all died for the Protestant faith. For Foxe, the most obvious ways to declare one's Protestant faith was to deny the doctrine of transubstantiation, refuse to participate in the Catholic church service, and refute Catholicism in theological debates. The Eusebian-style martyrs were useful for Foxe in depicting his martyrs as they faced the stake: Foxe could describe his martyrs as suffering patiently and heroically for the Protestant faith, just as Eusebius' martyrs suffered various tortures for their faith. However, the Eusebian-style martyrs were too taciturn if they were to be Foxe's models in any of the pre-execution scenes; Foxe needed his martyrs to be eloquent advocates of Protestantism, not merely silent sufferers. Thus, the Eusebian strength-within-weakness model was only used to describe female martyrs' behaviour in the torture and execution scenes of Rose Allin's martyrdom. The other elements of the story are informed by medieval hagiography instead.

She 'began to waxe weery of [th]e world': Joyce Lewis and Renunciation

In his account of Joyce Lewis's martyrdom, Foxe marks the woman's lifestyle change: 'Maistresse Ioyce Lewes, a gentlewoman borne, was delicately brought vp in the pleasures of [th]e world hauing delight in gay apparell & such like foolishness'.[70] John Glover, one highly respected Protestant, urged her to turn away from the Catholic Church and give up her love of worldly joys. With his advice in mind, Joyce Lewis 'began to waxe weery of [th]e world throughly sorrowfull for her sinnes, being inflamed with the loue of God, desirous to serue him accordyng to hys word, purposing also to flee from those thinges the whiche did displease the Lord her God'.[71]

The trope of the high-born woman renouncing her worldly pleasures for the sake of God is rarely, if ever, found in Eusebius. Eusebius categorised his female martyrs according to marriage status and age. Apart from Blandina, who was a slave, Eusebius did

---

[70] Foxe, *Acts and Monuments*, 2036.
[71] Foxe, *Acts and Monuments*, 2036.

not mention the social status of any female martyr whom he described in detail.[72] The reason for this was that Eusebius' martyrs tended to come from lower social classes and thus had little, aside from their lives, to give up.[73]

The surrender of worldly possessions as a holy act originates in the New Testament. For example, Jesus taught a rich man who came to him about how he might obtain eternal life: 'If thou wilt be perfect, go and sell that thou hast, and give to the poor, and thou shalt have treasure in heaven: and come and follow me'.[74] When the rich man departed sorrowfully, Jesus commented, 'it is easier for a camel to go through the eye of a needle, than for a rich man to enter into the kingdom of God'.[75] This and other teachings were followed literally by the desert hermits of the Eastern Church from the third century onward when the desert fathers established their sanctity through their understanding of God's words, asceticism, and complete renunciation of worldly pleasures and wealth. Some of the most noteworthy examples include St Antony in Athanasius' *Life of St Antony*[76] and the desert fathers in the *Apophthegmata Patrum*, or *Sayings of the Desert Fathers*.[77] Though

[72] Eusebius, *Ecclesiastical History*, volume 1, 415.
[73] For a discussion of the social background of Eusebius' martyrs compared with those of Foxe, see Freeman, '"Great searching out of bookes and autors"', 182-83. For a discussion of the mostly aristocratic background of medieval saints, see Katherine George and Charles H. George, 'Roman Catholic Sainthood', *Journal of Religion*, 5 (1953-55), 87; Alexander Murray, *Reason and Society in the Middle Ages* (Oxford, 1978), 337-41, 405-12; Donald Weinstein and Rudolph Bell, *Saints & Society: The Two Worlds of Western Christendom, 1000-1700* (Chicago, 1982), 196-99; Rodney Stark, 'Upper class asceticism: social origins of ascetic movements and medieval saints', *Review of Religious Research*, 45.1 (2003), 5-19. For a discussion of the social background of Foxe's martyrs, see Claire Cross, *The Church and People: England, 1450-1660* (Oxford, 1999), 113.
[74] Matthew 19:21.
[75] Matthew 19:24.
[76] Athanasius, 'Apophthegmata patrum, or Sayings of the Desert Fathers', in Nicene and Post-Nicene Fathers, second series, volume 4, edited by Philip Schaff and Henry Wace. Available from http://www.fordham.edu/Halsall/basis/vita-antony.asp [accessed 1 January 2011].
[77] The Sayings were originally passed on orally in Coptic, before being written down in the late fourth century. From the fifth and sixth centuries the Sayings were also translated into other languages such as Greek, Ethiopic, and Latin. In the seventeenth century, Heribert Rosweyde translated all of

some came from wealthy families, and others from more modest backgrounds, they all adopted a similar route to sanctity: the saints gave up their wealth to live in usually the Egyptian or Syrian deserts, fasted, prayed, practiced asceticism, fought monsters (real or imaginary) in the desert, and eventually became saints.[78] For example, St Antony's parents were 'of good family and possessed considerable wealth'. His parents brought him up in 'moderate affluence' but he never troubled his parents for 'luxurious fare' and was 'content simply with what he found nor sought anything further'.[79] When his parents died, he had a small sum saved for his younger sister. However, when he went to Church and heard again the passage, 'Be not anxious for the morrow', he gave up what little he had as well.[80] Worldly treasures were not only discarded but even detested in desert literature. When Melania the Elder, a fourth-century Roman aristocratic lady who did a grand tour of the Holy Land, gave three hundred pounds of gold to Pambo, a desert hermit, he instructed his steward to distribute the money to the poor. Melania anticipated some praise from him but the hermit only told her to keep quiet.[81]

By the time of Melania the Elder, Jerome, Ambrose, and Augustine, that is, the late fourth and early fifth centuries, the desert asceticism of the Greek East had become popular among the Roman elite in the Latin West, especially in Rome.[82] Since there

---

the Sayings into Latin and published them as the *Vitae patrum*. The first complete English translation was by Benedicta Ward. Benedicta Ward, *The Sayings of the Desert Fathers* (Kalamazoo, Michigan, 1975).

[78] For a discussion of gender in desert literature, see Anne Clark Bartlett, *Male Authors, Female Readers: Representation and Subjectivity in Middle English Devotional Literature* (Ithaca and London, 1995), 37-40.

[79] Athanasius, *Life of St Antony*, Chapter 1, 196.

[80] Athanasius, *Life of St Antony*, Chapter 3, 196.

[81] Palladius, *Historica lausiaca*, Chapter 46, 'Melania the Elder'. The English translation is available from http://www.fordham.edu/halsall/basis/palladius-lausiac.asp [accessed 1 January 2011].

[82] For excerpts from early Christian and patristic texts on asceticism, see Elizabeth Clark, *Message of the Fathers of the Church*, volume 13, edited by Thomas Halton (Collegeville, US, 1983), 115-55. For discussions of the patristic fathers' views toward women and female asceticism in the early Christian and patristic period, see Gillian Cloke, *'This Female Man of God': Women and Spiritual Power in the Patristic Age, AD 350-450* (London and New York, 1995); Lynda L. Coon, *Sacred Fictions: Holy Women and*

was no desert to retreat to, these 'urban desert saints' focused on the aspects of desert asceticism that they could manage to achieve, namely, relinquishing wealth, renouncing sexual activities, and practising asceticism.

Since much scholarship has been conducted on early Christian desert asceticism and its influence on the Church Fathers, I will focus on St Jerome, since he dealt extensively with female asceticism.[83] Jerome established protocols for his disciples (usually aristocratic women) to follow, and reinforced the concept that renouncing wealth was the first step to achieving sanctity.[84] Following the death of Paula, Jerome penned a letter to Paula's daughter, Eustochium, who was also an ascetic. In this letter, which is also a *vita* of Paula, Jerome describes how prominent Paula's family was since Paula's mother was descended from the Scipios and the Gracchi and her father from the line of Agamemnon. However, she still relinquished her wealth and title to live an ascetic life.[85] When she took a grand tour of the Holy Land just as Melania the Elder did before her, she 'rode upon an ass though as a noble woman, she was used to being carried by eunuchs'.[86] As an ascetic

---

Hagiography in Late Antiquity (Philadelphia, 1997); Susanna Elm, *'Virgins of God': The Making of Asceticism in Late Antiquity* (Oxford, 1994).

[83] Elizabeth Clark, *Jerome, Chrysostom, and Friends: Essays and Translations*, Studies in Women and Religion, volume 2 (New York and Toronto, 1979); Peter Brown, *The Body and Society: Men, Women, and Sexual Renunciation in Early Christianity* (New York, 1988); *That Gentle Strength: Historical Perspectives on Women in Christianity*, edited by Lynda L. Coon, Katherine J. Haldane, and Elisabeth W. Sommer (Charlottesville and London, 1990) and Kim Haines-Eitzen, *The Gendered Palimpsest: Women, Writing, and Representation in Early Christianity* (Oxford, 2012).

[84] More specifically on Jerome's attitude towards asceticism, see Andrew Cain, *The Letters of Jerome: Asceticism, Biblical Exegesis, and the Construction of Christian Authority in Late Antiquity* (Oxford, 2009); and Andrew Cain, 'Jerome's *Epitaphium Paulae*: hagiography, pilgrimage, and the cult of Saint Paula', *Journal of Early Christian Studies*, 18.1 (2010), 105-39.

[85] Jerome, Epistle 108.2-3, *Jerome: Letters and Select Works*, translated by William H. Freemantle, in Nicene and Post-Nicene Fathers, second series, volume 6, edited by Philip Schaff and Henry Wace (Edinburgh, 1893). The text can be found online in the Christian Classics Ethereal Library: http://www.ccel.org/ccel/schaff/npnf206.html [accessed 10 July 2013].

[86] Jerome, *Epistle*, 108.7.

living in Bethlehem, she was 'always the least remarkable in dress, in speech, in gesture, and in gait'.[87]

Though the trope of renouncing worldly wealth as a sign of sanctity originates in the writings of the Church Fathers, it remained accessible to later writers, including Foxe, through the *Golden Legend*. The saints featured in the *Golden Legend* share some characteristics with their early Christian and patristic predecessors in their renunciation of worldly pleasures and in their aristocratic status. However, there are still major differences. While some ascetic early saints do experience miraculous events, their *vitae* usually focus on their asceticism and especially sexual renunciation but not the saints' miracle-working abilities.[88]

On the other hand, the saints in the *Golden Legend* typically do not become ascetics; instead, they become wonder-workers. The female saints in the *Golden Legend* are usually virgin martyrs who work wonders to demonstrate God's (and their) power and to preserve their virginity. The legends of virgin martyrs follow a general pattern: the saint rejects her worldly possessions, refuses the marriage proposal of a wealthy, powerful suitor, and eventually sacrifices her life for her virginity and faith. For example, in St Agnes' legend, the prefect's son fell in love with her and offered her great wealth if she would consent to marry him. She refused and his father, finding out the reason for his son's lovesickness, offered even more wealth to Agnes. Agnes, in refusing the prefect, described the great wealth that Christ had already offered her.[89] Agnes later survived several rounds of torture miraculously.

When we compare virgin martyrs with their predecessors in ascetic literature, we discover that both virgin martyrs and ascetic

---

[87] Jerome, *Epistle*, 108.15.

[88] For example, Athanasius does not place too much emphasis on St Antony's miracle-working power but more on his battles with the demons in the desert and his Christian mission. Gorgonia in Gregory Nazianzus' *vita* of Gorgonia is said to have recovered miraculously from a carriage accident but the incident is depicted to demonstrate Gorgonia's feminine modesty rather than her miracle-working ability. See Gregory Nazianzus, 'On his sister Gorgonia', section 15, 242-43, in *Select Orations, Sermons, Letters; Dogmatic Treatises*, Nicene and Post-Nicene Fathers, second series, volume 7, edited by Philip Schaff and Henry Wace (reprinted Grand Rapids, US, 1955), VII.

[89] Voragine, *Golden Legend*, volume 1, 102.

saints see sexual renunciation as one of the most important elements of the renunciation of worldly pleasures. However, while in ascetic literature, sexual renunciation leads to an ascetic life, in virgin martyr legends, sexual renunciation leads to a miracle-working career. Returning to Joyce Lewis, Foxe described her as someone who had voluntarily relinquished worldly vanity. We cannot be sure which models Joyce Lewis' Protestant teacher, John Glover, had in mind when he advised her to give up worldly vanities but we can at least know for sure that he did not see Eusebius' early Christian martyrs as models of renunciation since these martyrs had few 'worldly vanities' to give up. Aristocratic saints in ascetic literature and the *Golden Legend* seem to be more likely models for Joyce Lewis.

However, John Foxe carved out a Protestant mode of renunciation for Joyce Lewis, rather than following earlier models of renunciation to the letter. Lewis was initially inspired by the martyrdom of Laurence Saunders, a prominent Protestant preacher burned in 1555. She 'enquired earnestly ... [the] cause of hys death'.[90] When she discovered it was because 'hee refused to receaue the Masse, she began to be troubled in conscie[n]ce & waxed very vnquiet' and asked John Glover to teach her 'the faultes that were in the Masse, and other things that at that time were vrged as necessary to saluation'.[91] John Glover 'most dilligently instruct[ed] her' that 'the Masse, with all other papisticall inuentions, was odious in Gods sight'.[92] He then 'reproued her, for that she delighted in the vanities of this world so much'.[93] By adding renunciation of 'the vanities of this world' to his advice against 'papisticall inuentions', John Glover aligned these with the Catholic Church and Protestantised a long tradition of renunciation present in biblical and ascetic literature, and medieval hagiography.

After Joyce Lewis renounced worldly vanities, she did not continue to live an ascetic and celibate life as did the desert saints, nor did she work miracles like the saints in the *Golden Legend*.

---

[90] Foxe, *Acts and Monuments*, 2036.
[91] Foxe, *Acts and Monuments*, 2036.
[92] Foxe, *Acts and Monuments*, 2036.
[93] Foxe, *Acts and Monuments*, 2036.

Instead, Foxe placed her directly at the centre of the struggles between Protestant and Catholic theology. Joyce Lewis's Protestant leaning eventually attracted the attention of the Catholic authorities, and despite her husband's strong protests, she was examined and encouraged to submit to the Catholic faith. The bishop released her the first time because she was a gentlewoman, and her husband was charged to bring her back after a month for a reexamination. However, Joyce Lewis showed no sign of committing to the Catholic faith, and even John Glover began to fear that she was seeking a martyr's death. In her second examination, she was sentenced to burning. On the eve of her execution, Joyce Lewis oscillated between joy and fear in her prison cell, but come morning, with the encouragement of her friends and supporters, she faced her burning courageously.[94] As we have seen in Rose Allin's account, Foxe only used the Eusebian model when he was depicting his martyrs' resolution in torture and death. Similarly, Joyce Lewis died in the manner of Eusebian martyrs, yet her renunciation of worldly vanities was most likely drawn from ascetic literature and medieval hagiography.

He 'called me in my bed, & at midnight opened his truth to me': Mrs Prest and Mysticism

Mrs Prest was the wife of a man named Prest and a mother of several children. When her husband forced her to conform to the Catholic faith, she left him and her children and supported herself financially by spinning. When she was examined, she replied, 'where I must either forsake Christ, or my husband, I am conte[n]ted to sticke onely to Christ my heauenly spouse, and renounce the other'.[95] She exhorted Daniel, a Protestant preacher during King Edward's reign, who recanted during Mary's reign, to repent. She also impressed the wife of Walter Rauley with her knowledge of Scripture and her godly talk. The wife of Walter Rauley declared to her husband that 'she neuer heard a woman (of such simplicity to see to) talk so godly, so perfectly, so sincerely, & so earnestly: in so muche that if God were not with her, shee could

[94] Foxe, *Acts and Monuments*, 2036-37.
[95] Foxe, *Acts and Monuments*, 2074.

not speak such things', especially since Mrs Prest was an illiterate woman.[96]

In Mrs Prest's examination, she argued with the Catholic doctors and bishops in such a learned way that the Catholics concluded that she must either have been taught by a Protestant preacher or be a mad woman. They tried hard to place her back in the domestic realm and ordered her husband to take her home but she refused to go. In their second examination, the authorities ridiculed her answers. An old friar asked her what she thought of the holy Pope and she replied that 'he is Antichrist and the deuill', much to the mirth of the examiners.[97] If Mrs Prest had left it at that, she might have gotten away with it. However, she pressed on and said, 'nay (sayde she) you had more neede to weepe then to laugh, & to be sory that euer you were borne, to be the chapleines of that whore of Babilon. I defie him and all hys falshood: and get you away fro[m] me: you do but trouble my conscience. You would haue me folow your doinges: I will first loose my life. I pray you depart'.[98] She then lectured the Catholic doctors on idolatry, purgatory, confession, and other 'Catholic abominations'. When the humour ran out, she was called 'an Anabaptist, a madde woman, a drunkard, a whoore, a runnagate'.[99] Finally, when asked again how she came to her opinion, she expressed that she had direct access to God and that she learned this from the one who 'called [her] in [her] bed, & at midnight opened his truth to [her]', and there was 'a great shout and laughing among the priestes and other'.[100]

The story of Mrs Prest has received extensive treatment in Megan Hickerson's *Making Women Martyrs in Tudor England*.[101] Hickerson situates Mrs Prest within the wider context of Foxe's concept of the Two Churches, that is, the True or Protestant Church and the False or Catholic Church. In Hickerson's analysis, Mrs Prest, stating that she must forsake her earthly husband in

---

[96] Foxe, *Acts and Monuments*, 2075.
[97] Foxe, *Acts and Monuments*, 2075.
[98] Foxe, *Acts and Monuments*, 2075.
[99] Foxe, *Acts and Monuments*, 2075.
[100] Foxe, *Acts and Monuments*, 2075.
[101] Hickerson, *Making Women Martyrs*.

favour of her heavenly husband, Christ, is read as a Bride of Christ. Hickerson also claims that this Bride of Christ is a group made up of male and female individuals and that though the individuals might behave in problematic ways, the collective Bride of Christ stood for the Protestant faith. For Hickerson, being the Bride of Christ justified a woman's decision to leave her husband because she was a member of the True Church. Yet, there is an alternative reading of the way in which John Foxe utilised the Bride of Christ image.

Mrs Prest's mystical midnight experience and her claim that she had to forsake her earthly husband for her heavenly husband, Christ, echoes the mystical marriages of female saints to Christ, found in the *Golden Legend*. One of the most famous unions can be found in the legend of St Katherine. The author states that Katherine was called unto baptism 'in a special manner' and that she 'was visibly married to our Lord'.[102] In this story, the Virgin Mary appeared to a holy desert hermit named Adrian and asked him to bring Katherine to the desert so that she could 'have [Christ] to her everlasting spouse'. When Adrian and Katherine entered the desert, a magnificent monastery suddenly appeared, waiting inside were the Virgin Mary and Christ. Mary wedded Katherine to Christ. As soon as Katherine heard Christ utter her name, 'so great a sweetness entered into her soul that she was all ravished'. Christ placed a ring upon her finger and bade her farewell. Katherine fell in a swoon for sorrow that Christ had departed. When Adrian finally revived her, she discovered that she was in an old cell and the grand monastery was nowhere to be seen. However, she found that the ring was still on her finger and drew much comfort from it. After this episode, she faced persecution bravely and eventually died a martyr's death.

When Foxe's story of Mrs Prest and the legend of St Katherine in the *Golden Legend* are examined in conjunction, we discover a Protestantised Bride of Christ. Though the Bride of Christ topos was replete with many Catholic connotations, such as the emphasis

---

[102] Jacobus de Voragine, 'The Life of Katherine', in *The Golden Legend*, edited by Frederick S. Ellis (Edinburgh, 1900). Accessible online at: http://www.fordham.edu/halsall/basis/goldenlegend/GoldenLegend-Volume7.asp#Katherine [accessed 10 July 2013].

on virginity and the mystical and somewhat erotic union between a female saint and Christ, Foxe did not simply discard the topos. Instead, he Protestantised it and used this commonly known bridal rhetoric to his advantage. When Mrs Prest stated that she had been taught by someone who 'called [her] in [her] bed, & at midnight opened his truth to [her]', Foxe was probably evoking the powerful image of St Katherine and other famous Brides of Christ and transforming Mrs Prest into a potent Protestantised Bride of Christ.

Conclusion

This analysis of the accounts of three female martyrs described by John Foxe challenges the notion in mainstream Reformation scholarship that Foxe only derived his models for female martyrs from early Christian martyrologies and more specifically, from Eusebius. Though it is apparent that Foxe did indeed draw inspiration from early Christian materials as he claimed, there is much to glean if we do not accept at face value Foxe's statement that he detested the *Golden Legend* so greatly that he would never have anything to do with it. From the case studies of Rose Allin, Joyce Lewis, and Mrs Prest, we can conclude that, though Foxe claimed he distanced himself from popish superstitions and outlandish miracles, he was more accepting of medieval hagiography than he admitted. Indeed, in many ways Foxe was as equally influenced by medieval hagiography as he was by Eusebius. Foxe's female martyrs can be considered just as much descendants of Voragine's saints as they were of Eusebius' martyrs. However, even when Foxe utilised hagiographical themes and rhetoric normally associated with the *Golden Legend*, he presented a Protestantised version of a female martyr. Though we cannot know for sure which models of behaviour Foxe or his female martyrs themselves had in mind, this comparison of Foxe's depictions of female martyrs with those presented in early Christian martyrology and medieval hagiographical texts reveals his use of earlier methods for demonstrating sanctity in terms of verbal defence of the true faith, divine analgesia, renunciation of worldly vanities, and a mystical union with Christ. Foxe's female martyrs exhibited more traditional models of sanctity than has previously been assumed, though reshaped into a Protestantised mould. This chapter has offered a new approach to reading Foxe's *Acts and Monuments*, emphasising the continuities between pre- and post-Reformation depictions of saints and martyrs.

THE CONTRIBUTORS

Anne E. Bailey completed her doctorate in July 2010, and from 2010-2013 held a postdoctoral research fellowship at Harris Manchester College, University of Oxford. She is currently researching and teaching at Oxford where she is affiliated to the History Faculty. Her research interests include saints' cults and pilgrimage, hagiography, women's religious history, and medical history, focusing primarily on England during the high middle ages.

Kati Ihnat is currently a postdoctoral researcher at the University of Bristol where she is working on religious culture in early medieval Spain. She completed her PhD at Queen Mary, University of London, and went on to take up fellowships at Trinity College Dublin and the University of Pennsylvania. Her research focuses on the history of religious practice from an interdisciplinary perspective that includes liturgy, sermons, theological polemic and miracle literature.

Fiona Kao is doing her PhD in Divinity at Cambridge (expected 2015). She is working on John Foxe's female martyrs in the Acts and Monuments. She looks at how Foxe utilises pre-existing tropes in early Christian, patristic, and medieval hagiographical texts in presenting his Protestant female martyrs.

Iona McCleery has been Lecturer in Medieval History at the University of Leeds since 2007. She was previously Wellcome fellow in the History of Medicine at the University of Durham. Her research focuses on the history of healthcare, food and healing in the late Middle Ages, especially in Portugal. Her Ph.D. thesis from the University of St Andrews (2000) focused on the life of St Gil de Santarém. She ran the Wellcome Trust funded project *You Are What You Ate: Food Lessons from the Past* in 2010-2014 (www.leeds.ac.uk/youarewhatyouate). Recent publications include essays on the female patient, medical licensing and King Duarte of Portugal's (d. 1438) attitude towards dietary regimen. Future work will explore the impact of Portuguese colonialism on diet and medicine in the late middle ages with forthcoming essays on travel and famine.

Matthew Mesley is a postdoctoral Research Assistant at the University of Zurich, and is part of a research project which is funded by the Swiss National Science Foundation. His research focuses predominately upon bishops and the ways in which gender ideals influenced episcopal activity within the political sphere. For the academic year 2013-4, he was awarded Senior Membership at Robinson College, Cambridge and was a visiting fellow at the Center for Medieval Studies at Fordham University, New York. Recent publications include 'Episcopal authority and gender in the narratives of the First Crusade', in *Religious Men and Masculine Identity in the Middle Ages*, edited by P. Cullum and K. J. Lewis (Boydell and Brewer: Woodbridge, 2013) and '"De Judaea, muta et surda": Jewish conversion in Gerald of Wales's *Life of Saint Remigius*', in *Christians and Jews in Angevin England: The York Massacre of 1190, Narratives and Contexts*, edited by Sarah Rees Jones and Sethina Watson (York Medieval Press: York, 2013).

Irina Metzler works on the cultural, religious and social aspects of physical disability in the European middle ages. She has combined the approaches of modern Disability Studies with historical sources to investigate the intellectual framework within which medieval cultures positioned physically impaired persons. A second monograph on social and economic conditions of medieval disability was published in 2013. Her current project examines notions of intellectual impairment in the middle ages. Dr Metzler's wider research interests revolve around medieval notions of history and the past, perceptions of the natural world (in particular cats as ambiguous animals), and historical anthropology. Irina Metzler gained her PhD from the University of Reading in 2001 and joined the University of Swansea as a Wellcome Trust-funded Research Fellow in 2012.

Rebecca Pinner teaches in the School of Literature, Drama and Creative Writing at the University of East Anglia. Her primary research interests concern the relationship between literature, context and culture, the construction and dissemination of individual and collective identities and relationships between literature and other cultural artefacts. She has published several articles and chapters on these and related issues and her first book, on the cult of St Edmund in medieval East Anglia, will be published with Boydell and Brewer in 2015.

Louise Elizabeth Wilson is a Research Assistant at the University of Bristol and an Affiliated Scholar with the Department of History and Philosophy of Science at the University of Cambridge. Her research focuses on the history of the natural and supernatural in medieval Europe, examining the interactions between medical, natural philosophical and theological ideas. She is currently writing a monograph about witchcraft, harmful magic and medicine in medieval England, exploring the attitudes of medical practitioners to hostile magic, the impact of developments in Christian theology on these attitudes and the role played by physicians and other practitioners of medicine in the prosecutions of hostile magic and witchcraft.

Simon Yarrow is Senior Lecturer in Medieval History at the University of Birmingham. His primary research is on the cult of saints in the Medieval West from the eleventh to the thirteenth centuries. His monograph, *Saints and Their Communities, Miracle Narratives in Twelfth-Century England* came out with OUP in 2006, and he has written further articles on the cult of saints and pilgrimage, and on twelfth-century English chronicles with particular attention to religious piety, ethnic and religious identities, and gender. He has recently published on the topic of masculinity and world history, and on the value of anthropology to historians of medieval Christianity. Simon belongs to the 'Social Church Group' who are currently working on new approaches to the history of medieval Christianity for research and teaching purposes. He also belongs to the steering committee of the 'Global Middle Ages' research network.